HERBS

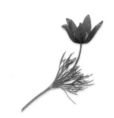

HERBS

A color guide to herbs
and herbal healing

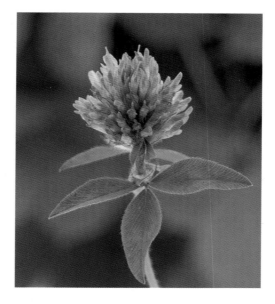

JENNIE HARDING

CHARTWELL
BOOKS

Inspiring | Educating | Creating | Entertaining

Brimming with creative inspiration, how-to projects, and useful information to enrich your everyday life, Quarto Knows is a favorite destination for those pursuing their interests and passions. Visit our site and dig deeper with our books into your area of interest: Quarto Creates, Quarto Cooks, Quarto Homes, Quarto Lives, Quarto Drives, Quarto Explores, Quarto Gifts, or Quarto Kids.

This edition published in 2017 by Chartwell Books
an imprint of The Quarto Group
142 West 36th Street, 4th Floor
New York, New York 10018, USA
T (212) 779-4972 F (212) 779-6058
www.QuartoKnows.com

First published in the UK in 2007

Chartwell Books titles are also available at discount for retail, wholesale, promotional, and bulk purchase. For details, contact the Special Sales Manager by email at specialsales@quarto.com or by mail at The Quarto Group, Attn: Special Sales Manager, 401 Second Avenue North, Suite 310, Minneapolis, MN 55401, USA.

10 9 8 7 6 5 4 3 2 1

ISBN-13: 978-0-7858-3568-4

Printed in China

This book was conceived, designed, and produced by
Ivy Press
an imprint of The Quarto Group
6 Blundell Street, London N7 9BH, UK

Creative Director Peter Bridgewater
Publisher Jason Hook
Editorial Director Caroline Earle
Art Director Clare Harris
Senior Project Editor James Thomas
Designer Ginny Zeal
Concept Design Alan Osbahr
Picture Research Katie Greenwood, Shelley Noronha

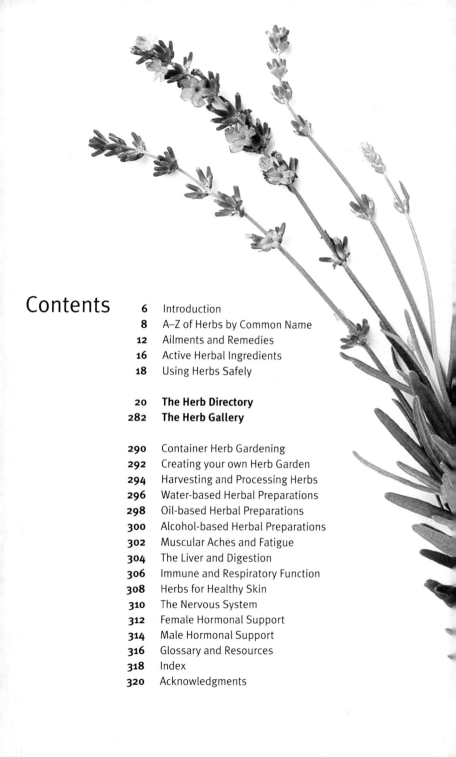

Contents

6   Introduction
8   A–Z of Herbs by Common Name
12 Ailments and Remedies
16 Active Herbal Ingredients
18 Using Herbs Safely

20 **The Herb Directory**
282 **The Herb Gallery**

290 Container Herb Gardening
292 Creating your own Herb Garden
294 Harvesting and Processing Herbs
296 Water-based Herbal Preparations
298 Oil-based Herbal Preparations
300 Alcohol-based Herbal Preparations
302 Muscular Aches and Fatigue
304 The Liver and Digestion
306 Immune and Respiratory Function
308 Herbs for Healthy Skin
310 The Nervous System
312 Female Hormonal Support
314 Male Hormonal Support
316 Glossary and Resources
318 Index
320 Acknowledgments

INTRODUCTION

Herbs—medicinal plants with special healing properties—have always played an important part in human history, cultural development, and experience. Since prehistoric times, particular plants have been favored not just as foods or flavorings, but also because of their medicinal effects. Every culture on the planet has its own traditional remedies made from local plants, using particular leaves, roots, or flowers for their specific health benefits. For centuries before written records, herb knowledge was passed on orally from generation to generation.

HERBS IN HISTORY

The medical use of herbs can be traced back in the history of many ancient civilizations. In China, a famous 4,000-year-old text, *The Yellow Emperor's Book of Internal Medicine*, recorded remedies such as ginger for helping the digestion, and opium for relieving pain. The Indian tradition of using herbs and spices goes back approximately 4,000 years to the Vedic texts, which form the basis for Ayurvedic medicine, in which aromatic ingredients such as cilantro, sandalwood, and pepper were used to balance the body, mind, and spirit. In early medieval times Arab civilization was renowned for its healing knowledge; Arab physician, Abu Ibn Sina (980–1037) is famous for his *Canon of Medicine*, a text that describes many medicinal plants such as camphor, camomile, and lavender.

Western herbal medicine stretches back to the ancient Greeks, who in turn learned from the ancient Egyptians. Hippocrates, born in Greece around 460 BCE, used herbs such as lungwort for lung infections. Another Greek physician—Dioscorides—cataloged all the plants and spices available in his time; his work, published in 78 CE, called *De Materia Medica*, remained a classic Western herbal text for several centuries after his death.

The 16th and 17th centuries in England produced some of the most famous Western herbalists, such as John Gerard (1545–1611), who grew an incredible collection of herbs in his own garden in Holborn in London, and Nicholas Culpeper (1616–54) whose famous *Herbal* of 1649 made information on herbs and healing widely available.

HERBAL MEDICINE TODAY

Despite the development of chemical drugs during the 18th and 19th centuries and the preeminence of the pharmaceutical companies in the 20th and 21st centuries, herbal medicine has survived and is enjoying renewed popularity, since it offers a more natural way to maintain health and well-being. Today, professional herbalists still use traditional preparations such as dried herbs, infusions, tinctures, and ointments with their clients. Many herbs are now being researched using modern scientific methods, which often confirm their efficacy and traditional applications.

This book is intended as a detailed introduction to the world of herbs and healing. It is designed as a practical guide to choosing and using herbs sensibly and safely to support health. As we shall see, although herbs and herbal remedies are "natural," this does not mean they can be used freely; many are very potent and need to be used carefully. Individual profiles of 130 herbs in the extensive Herb Directory (pages 20–281) will give you a wide range to choose from for different problems and conditions. Later you will find a lovely Herb Gallery with illustrations of all featured herbs (pages 282–288) followed by several sections of practical suggestions and guidelines to help you to absorb the healing properties of herbs into your life.

A–Z OF HERBS BY COMMON NAME

Below is a list of all of the herbs contained within the Herb Directory, listed alphabetically according to their common name, alongside their Latin name and the page number on which they appear within the Directory.

Agnus castus	*Vitex agnus castus*	276
Aloe vera	*Aloe vera*	30
Angelica	*Angelica archangelica*	36
Arnica	*Arnica montana*	52
Basil	*Ocimum basilicum*	178
Bay laurel	*Laurus nobilis*	148
Bearberry [uva ursi]	*Arctostaphylos uva ursi*	48
Betony [wood]	*Stachys officinalis*	238
Birch, silver	*Betula pendula*	60
Black cohosh	*Cimifuga racemosa*	74
Blackcurrant	*Ribes nigrum*	206
Borage	*Borago officinalis*	62
Burdock	*Arctium lappa*	46
Calendula	*Calendula officinalis*	66
Camomile, Roman	*Anthemis nobilis*	40
Camomile, German	*Matricaria chamomilla*	164
Cardamom	*Elettaria cardamomum*	100
Carrot	*Daucus carota*	94
Cayenne pepper	*Capsicum frutescens*	68
Celery seed	*Apium graveolens*	44
Centaury	*Erythrea centaurium*	106
Chervil	*Anthriscus cerefolium*	42
Cilantro	*Coriandrum sativum*	86
Cinnamon	*Cinnamomum zeylanicum*	76
Clary sage	*Salvia scalrea*	222
Clove	*Eugenia caryophylla*	110
Coltsfoot	*Tussilago farfara*	260
Comfrey	*Symphytum officinale*	240
Cornflower	*Centaurea cyanus*	72

Cowslip	*Primula veris*	200
Cranberry	*Vaccinium macrocarpon*	266
Daisy	*Bellis perennis*	58
Damiana	*Turnera diffusa*	258
Dandelion	*Taraxum officinale*	246
Devil's claw	*Harpogophytum procumbens*	132
Dill	*Anethum graveolens*	34
Dong quai	*Angelica polymorpha*	38
Echinacea	*Echinacea purpurea*	98
Elder	*Sambucus nigra*	224
Eucalyptus	*Eucalyptus globules*	108
Evening primrose	*Oenothera biennis*	180
Eyebright	*Euphrasia officinalis*	112
Fennel	*Foeniculum vulgare*	116
Fenugreek	*Trigonella foenum-graecum*	254
Feverfew	*Tanacetum parthenium*	244
Garlic	*Allium sativum*	28
Ginger	*Zingiber officinale*	280
Gingko	*Gingko biloba*	126
Ginseng	*Panax ginseng*	188
Golden rod	*Solidago virgauerea*	236
Golden seal	*Hydrastis canadensis*	140
Grapefruit	*Citrus paradisi*	82
Grapeseed extract	*Vitis vinifera*	278
Hawthorn	*Crategus oxyacantha*	88
Heather	*Erica vulgaris*	104
Hops	*Humulus lupulus*	138
Horehound [white]	*Marrulum vulgare*	162
Horse chestnut	*Aesculus hippocastanum*	24
Horseradish	*Armoracia rusticana*	50
Horsetail fern	*Equisetum arvense*	102
Hyssop	*Hyssopus officinalis*	144
Juniper	*Juniperus communis*	146
Kava kava	*Piper methrysticum*	196

Kelp/bladderwrack	*Fucus vesiculosus*	120
Lady's bedstraw	*Galium verum*	122
Lady's mantle	*Alchemilla vulgaris*	26
Lavender	*Lavandula angustifolia*	150
Lemon	*Citrus limonum*	80
Lemon verbena	*Lippia citriodora*	158
Lemongrass	*Cymbopogon citratus*	92
Licorice	*Glycyrrhiza glabra*	128
Linden/ lime flower	*Tilia cordata*	250
Lobelia	*Lobelia inflata*	160
Lovage	*Levisticum officinale*	156
Lungwort	*Pulmonaria officinalis*	202
Manuka	*Leptospermum scoparium*	154
Marjoram	*Origanum marjorana*	184
Meadowsweet	*Filipendula ulmaria*	114
Melissa	*Melissa officinalis*	168
Milk thistle	*Silybum marianum*	234
Motherwort	*Leonurus cardiaca*	152
Mulberry	*Morus nigra*	174
Mullein	*Verbascum thapsus*	270
Mustard seeds [black]	*Brassica nigra*	64
Myrrh	*Commiphora myrrha*	84
Myrtle	*Myrtus communis*	176
Nasturtium	*Tropaeolum majus*	256
Nettle	*Urtica diotica*	264
Oak	*Quercus robur*	204
Oat	*Avena sativa*	56
Olive	*Olea europea*	182
Orange, bitter	*Citrus aurantium*	78
Oregano	*Origanum vulgare*	186
Parsley	*Petroselinum crispum*	192
Pasque flower	*Anemone pulsatilla*	32
Passion flower	*Passiflora incarnata*	190
Pau d'arco	*Tabebuia avellanedae*	242

Pepper, black	*Piper nigrum*	198
Peppermint	*Mentha x piperita*	172
Pine	*Pinus sylvestris*	194
Raspberry	*Rubea idaeus*	214
Red clover	*Trifolium pratense*	252
Rose	*Rosa damascena, Rosa gallica, Rosa centifolia*	210
Rose hips	*Rosa canina*	208
Rosemary	*Rosmarinus officinale*	212
Sage	*Salvia officinalis*	220
Savory	*Satureja hortensis*	228
Saw palmetto	*Serenoa serrulata*	232
Sea buckthorn	*Hippophae rhamnoides*	136
Senna	*Cassia senna*	70
Skullcap	*Scutellaria lateriflora*	230
Slippery elm	*Ulmus fulva*	262
Soapwort	*Saponaria officinalis*	226
Sorrel	*Rumex acetosa*	216
Spearmint	*Mentha spicata*	170
St. John's wort	*Hypericum perforatum*	142
Sunflower	*Helianthus annuus*	134
Tarragon	*Artemisis dracunculus*	54
Tea tree	*Melaeluca alternifolia*	166
Thyme	*Thymus vulgaris*	248
Turmeric	*Curcuma longa*	90
Valerian	*Valeriana officinalis*	268
Vervain	*Verbena officinalis*	272
White willow	*Salix alba*	218
Wild strawberry	*Fragaria vesca*	118
Wild violet	*Viola odorata*	274
Wild yam	*Dioscorea villosa*	96
Witch hazel	*Hamamelis virginiana*	130
Yarrow	*Achillea millefolium*	22
Yellow gentian	*Gentiana lutea*	124

AILMENTS AND REMEDIES

Below is a list of common ailments, alongside the various herbal remedies that can be used to treat them. The pages on which the herbs appear within the Herb Directory are included in brackets after each herb.

Age-related cognitive decline, Alzheimer's disease	Gingko (126), rosemary (212)
Anemia	Turmeric (90), horsetail fern (102), parsley (192), nettle (264)
Asthma	Gingko (126), licorice (128), sunflower (134)
Bladder and urinary tract infections, e.g., cystitis	Bearberry/uva ursi (48), silver birch (60), wild strawberry (118), lady's bedstraw (122), myrtle (176), parsley (192), blackcurrant (206), goldenrod (236), pau d'arco (242), dandelion (246), nasturtium (256), cranberry (266)
Bleeding	Yarrow (22), horsetail fern (102), lady's bedstraw (122), witch hazel (130)
Blocked sinuses	Eucalyptus (108), peppermint (172), basil (178)
Brittle nails, thinning hair	Horsetail fern (102)
Broken bones (first aid)	Comfrey (240)
Bruises, sprains	Arnica (52), daisy (58), witch hazel (130), St. John's wort (142), wood betony (238), comfrey (240), fenugreek (254), wild violet (274)
Burns (including radiation burns)	Aloe vera (30), sea buckthorn (136), St. John's wort (142), lavender (150), rose (210), comfrey (240), slippery elm (262)
Cold limbs, chilblains	Cayenne pepper (68), oak (204), rosemary (212), thyme (248), lime flower (250), ginger (280)
Cold sores, shingles [Herpes]	Melissa (168)
Colds	Yarrow (22), lemon (80), turmeric (90), echinacea (98), cardamom (100), eucalyptus (108), clove (110), bay laurel (148), manuka (154), tea tree (166), peppermint (172), mulberry (174), basil (178), pine (194), black pepper (198), blackcurrant (206), rose hip (208), sage (220), elder (224), saw palmetto (232), thyme (248), wild violet (274)
Colitis, irritable bowel syndrome	Aloe vera (30), dill (34), peppermint (172), fenugreek (254), slippery elm (262)
Constipation	Dill (34), silver birch (60), senna (70), Devil's claw (132), goldenseal (140), olive (182), black pepper (198), dandelion (246), vervain (272)
Convalescence	Ginseng (188), slippery elm (262), vervain (272)
Coughs, bronchitis	Angelica (36), horseradish (50), daisy (58), myrrh (84), turmeric (90), cardamom (100), eucalyptus (108), clove (110), eyebright (112), licorice

	(128), goldenseal (140), hyssop (144), manuka (154), white horehound (162), tea tree (166), myrtle (176), basil (178), pine (194), cowslip (200), lungwort (202), sage (220), elder (224), savory (228), thyme (248), red clover (252), nasturtium (256), mullein (270), wild violet (274), ginger (280)
Cuts, wounds, grazes	Yarrow (22), Lady's mantle (26), aloe vera (30), burdock (46), daisy (58), calendula (66), turmeric (90), echinacea (98), eucalyptus (108), lady's bedstraw (122), witch hazel (130), Devil's claw (132), St. John's wort (142), lavender (150), manuka (154), white horehound (162), tea tree (166), oregano (186), lungwort (202), sorrel (216), goldenrod (236), wood betony (238), red clover (252), slippery elm (262)
Diarrhea	Lady's mantle (26), meadowsweet (114), oak (204)
Digestive nausea	Yellow gentian (124), lemon verbena (158), peppermint (172), ginger (280)
Dry, sensitive skin	Borage (62), cornflower (72), sunflower (134), evening primrose (180), olive (182), blackcurrant (206), rose (210), elder (224)
Earache	Mullein (270)
Eczema, psoriasis, shingles	Aloe vera (30), burdock (46), calendula (66), German camomile (164), melissa (168), evening primrose (180), soapwort (226), goldenrod (236), red clover (252)
Emotional shock	Arnica (52)
Fevers	Centaury (106), spearmint (170), sorrel (216), white willow (218), lime flower (250)
Fluid retention, bloating	Celery seed (44), bearberry/uva ursi (48), carrot (94), heather (104), fennel (116), juniper (146), parsley (192), rose hip (208), sorrel (216), dandelion (246)
Fungal infections, athlete's foot, thrush (candida)	Garlic (28), cinnamon (76), grapefruit (82), myrrh (84), tea tree (166), pau d'arco (242)
Gastric ulceration	Licorice (128)
Hemorrhoids (piles)	Horse chestnut (24), witch hazel (130), oak (204), grapeseed (278)
Hay fever, allergic rhinitis	Eyebright (112), melissa (168), elder (224)
Headache, migraine, PMS headache	Pasque flower (32), black cohosh (74), meadowsweet (114), lavender (150), motherwort (152), lemon verbena (158), cowslip (200), white willow (218), skullcap (230), feverfew (244), valerian (268)
High blood pressure	Garlic (28), dong quai (38), hawthorn (88), motherwort (152), olive (182), passion flower (190)
Hives, skin itching, irritation, dandruff	Roman camomile (40), German camomile (164), nettle (264)
Indigestion, digestive cramps, wind	Lady's mantle (26), aloe vera (30), dill (34), angelica (36), Roman camomile (40), chervil (42), celery seed (44), horseradish (50), oat (56), daisy (58), borage (62), calendula (66), cayenne pepper (68), cinnamon (76), grapefruit (82), cilantro (86), turmeric (90),

	lemongrass (92), carrot (94), wild yam (96), cardamom (100), centaury (106), clove (110), meadowsweet (114), fennel (116), wild strawberry (118), yellow gentian (124), licorice (128), Devil's claw (132), hop (138), bay laurel (148), lovage (156), lemon verbena (158), melissa (168), spearmint (170), peppermint (172), basil (178), marjoram (184), parsley (192), black pepper (198), white willow (218), savory (228), wood betony (238), dandelion (246), lime flower (250), fenugreek (254), vervain (272), ginger (280)
Influenza, low immunity	Garlic (28), burdock (46), cayenne pepper (68), cinnamon (76), lemon (80), echinacea (98), cardamom (100), clove (110), sea buckthorn (136), bay laurel (148), manuka (154), lovage (156), tea tree (166), mulberry (174), olive (182), black pepper (198), blackcurrant (206), rose hip (208), sage (220), elder (224), saw palmetto (232), pau d'arco (242), lime flower (250), cranberry (266), ginger (280)
Insect bites and stings	Lady's mantle (26), hyssop (144), lavender (150), basil (178), savory (228)
Insomnia	Lady's mantle (26), Roman camomile (40), oat (56), carrot (94), hop (138), lavender (150), motherwort (152), German camomile (164), melissa (168), marjoram (184), oregano (186), passion flower (190), cowslip (200), skullcap (230), feverfew (244), valerian (268), vervain (272)
Irritability, mental stress or pressure	Hop (138), St. John's wort (142), German camomile (164), melissa (168), spearmint (170), cowslip (200), lime flower (250), damiana (258)
Late pregnancy, labor, slow flow of breastmilk, menopausal issues (hot flashes, mood swings, fluctuating hormone levels, tiredness)	Lady's mantle (26), dong quai (38), borage (62), black cohosh (74), wild yam (96), St. John's wort (142), motherwort (152), German camomile (164), evening primrose (180), marjoram (184), blackcurrant (206), raspberry leaf (214), sage (220), clary sage (222), agnus castus (276)
Liver and gallbladder problems, indigestion of fatty foods	Centaury (106), yellow gentian (124), Devil's claw (132), lemon verbena (158), white horehound (162), oregano (186), parsley (192), rose (210), milk thistle (234), wood betony (238), vervain (272)
Liver damage (e.g., via alcohol or drugs, high levels of cellular toxicity)	Milk thistle (234), grapeseed (278)
Low physical energy, physical tiredness	Ginseng (188), oak (204), rose hip (208), rosemary (212), fenugreek (254), damiana (258), vervain (272)
Male reproductive issues	Pasque flower (32), fenugreek (254), damiana (258)
Male sexual difficulties, low libido	Turmeric (90), ginseng (188), saw palmetto (232), damiana (258)
Mature skin	Borage (62), bitter orange (78), sunflower (134), myrtle (176), evening primrose (180), blackcurrant (206), rose (210)
Muscular aches and pains	Mustard seed (black) (64), cayenne pepper (68), cilantro (86), lemongrass (92), heather (104), eucalyptus (108), Devil's claw (132), juniper (146), bay laurel (148), lavender (150), peppermint (172), marjoram (184), oregano (186), pine (194), black pepper (198), rosemary (212), thyme (248), ginger (280)

Nervous stress, tension, depression	Oat (56), lemongrass (92), bitter orange (78), gingko (126), lavender (150), motherwort (152), melissa (168), ginseng (188), passion flower (190), cowslip (200), oak (204), rose (210), skullcap (230), lime flower (250), damiana (258), valerian (268), vervain (272)
Neuralgia, sciatica	St. John's wort (142)
Oily/combination skin	Bitter orange (78), lemon (80), wild strawberry (118), myrtle (176)
PMS, menstrual pain, irregular periods, hormone imbalance	Lady's mantle (26), pasque flower (32), dong quai (38), borage (62), black cohosh (74), wild yam (96), St. John's wort (142), white horehound (162), evening primrose (180), marjoram (184), blackcurrant (206), raspberry (214), clary sage (222), skullcap (230), goldenrod (236), feverfew (244), red clover (252), damiana (258), nettle (264), agnus castus (276)
Poor circulation	Silver birch (60), mustard seed (black) (64), cayenne pepper (68), hawthorn (88), cardamom (100), pine (194), grapeseed (278)
Poor memory or concentration	Gingko (126), rosemary (212)
Prostate problems	Horsetail fern (102), saw palmetto (232), goldenrod (236), nasturtium (256)
Rheumatism, arthritis, gout	Yarrow (22), angelica (36), celery seed (44), burdock (46), horseradish (50), silver birch (60), mustard seed (black) (64), cinnamon (76), wild yam (96), cardamom (100), heather (104), centaury (106), meadowsweet (114), kelp (120), Devil's claw (132), hyssop (144), juniper (146), lovage (156), peppermint (172), marjoram (184), oregano (186), parsley (192), pine (194), cowslip (200), blackcurrant (206), rose hip (208), white willow (218), soapwort (226), feverfew (244), dandelion (246), nettle (264), cranberry (266)
Sore eyes, inflamed eyes, minor eye infections	Cornflower (72), eyebright (112), goldenseal (140)
Sore gums, mouth ulcers, toothache	Tarragon (54), cornflower (72), myrrh (84), echinacea (98), clove (110), eyebright (112), fennel (116), goldenseal (140), tea tree (166), sage (220), wild violet (274)
Sore throats	Goldenseal (140), mulberry (174), raspberry (214), sorrel (216), thyme (248), nasturtium (256), wild violet (274)
Spots, acne, boils, infected wounds	Daisy (58), echinacea (98), witch hazel (130), Devil's claw (132), lavender (150), tea tree (166), soapwort (226), slippery elm (262), mullein (270)
Sunburn	Aloe vera (30), wild strawberry (118), sea buckthorn (136), rose (210)
Thyroid imbalance	Kelp (120)
Varicose veins, broken veins	Horse chestnut (24), calendula (66), witch hazel (130), manuka (154), comfrey (240), grapeseed (278)
Weight gain	Kelp (120)

ACTIVE HERBAL INGREDIENTS

Herbs are special plants; they contain particular active compounds known by chemical names, given to them after scientific analysis. Many modern drugs are derived from herbs, such as aspirin from willow (*Salix alba*), but these are synthetic and concentrated around one active ingredient. In herbal medicine, however, the whole plant is used to make a remedy, even if there are only a few active ingredients present, because all the other chemicals in the plant are considered to work together to balance the active constituents, helping to prevent any side effects.

COMMON ACTIVE INGREDIENTS IN HERBS

Alkaloids are the most powerful of all plant constituents; they often affect the nervous system. Many alkaloid-rich herbs are not suitable for home use; a mild example is borage.

Bitters are bitter-tasting compounds which increase the flow of digestive juices improving all aspects of absorption and elimination. They are found in herbs like yellow gentian or German camomile.

Tannins are substances that have a protective effect on the skin, shielding it against infection and helping to reduce inflammation. Examples of tannin-rich herbs are horsetail, elderflower, and raspberry leaf.

Glycosides are natural sugars found in many herbs, such as German camomile and basil.

Gums and resins are sticky substances which ooze out of cracks in tree bark, as is seen in the myrrh tree.

Mucilages are gel-like substances that cool, soothe, and protect the skin, as well as the delicate membranes of the digestive, respiratory, and urinary systems. Comfrey or aloe vera leaves are examples.

LEFT: Raspberry leaf (far left) contains high levels of tannins, while borage (left) is rich in alkaloids

RIGHT: Elderflower (top) is rich in flavonoids, while calendula (bottom) is a source of saponins

Saponins are ingredients that can produce a lather when mixed with water. Historically, saponin-rich herbs were used as skin washes, hair rinses, or antiseptic skin cleansers. Good examples are oats and calendula.

Flavonoids are ingredients mainly found in plant tissues with yellow or white pigments. They help the circulation, protect blood-vessel walls, and help reduce inflammation. Examples are St. John's wort, yarrow, and elderflower.

Volatile oils are found in specialized cells in leaves, flowers, roots, woods, fruit peel, and berries. They have a powerful aroma, and are usually extracted by distillation, after which they are called "essential oils" and are used in aromatherapy. Lavender or rosemary are examples. Volatile oils contain many constituents, such as coumarins, esters, ketones, and terpenes.

Vitamins and trace elements assist in building vitality and are essential to overall health. All herbs are rich in these.

The combinations of active ingredients in herbs correlate directly to their physical uses, as you will see from the individual herb profiles in the Directory (pages 20–281). In each profile, the active ingredients are listed, as well as the benefits and uses of the herb. This places a herb in context, and the more you investigate the Directory the more you will find certain ingredients recur. This will help you to become familiar with categories of herbs linked to particular groups of conditions, such as those listed on pages 12–15.

LEFT: Volatile oils can be extracted from herbs such as rosemary

USING HERBS SAFELY

In order to obtain the maximum benefit from using herbs it is very important to use them safely and correctly. Just because herbs are natural does not automatically mean they can be taken without care. There is a fine line between simply enjoying an herbal tea, for example, and then deciding to use that tea for a particular effect and drinking a lot more of it (so-called "self-medication"). There are some golden rules that you should always follow when you are thinking of choosing and taking herbs yourself, and some other guidelines you need to bear in mind.

GOLDEN RULES

If you are on *any kind* of medication from the doctor, *always* seek medical advice before starting to take herbal medications. You should never discontinue drug treatment without medical guidance. Also, some herbs can counteract or increase the activity of particular drugs; for example, garlic has an anticoagulant effect, thinning the blood, so if you were already on anticoagulant medication the effect would be increased. The individual herb profiles within the Directory (pages 20–281) will point out any known contraindications.

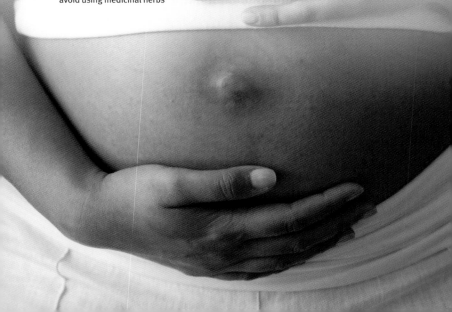

BELOW: If you are pregnant it is best to avoid using medicinal herbs

If you are feeling unwell or have any symptoms that you feel are unusual, you should always seek medical advice, and not attempt self-diagnosis.

If you are pregnant it is best to avoid using medicinal herbs at all unless you consult a professional herbalist for advice. Throughout the Directory all herbs that are specifically contraindicated for pregnancy are noted. However, as a rule of thumb, it is best to avoid all herbal remedies, especially for the first three months of pregnancy. Although some herbs, such as raspberry leaf, can help in labor, it is best to consult your midwife for guidance.

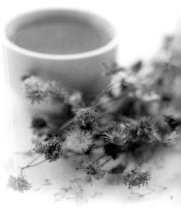

ABOVE: Safety is particularly important when taking herbs internally, for example in teas or infusions

METHODS OF USE

Safety is particularly important when it comes to taking herbs internally, for example when drinking infusions (herbal teas), swallowing tinctures or decoctions, or taking capsules or tablets. This is because the active ingredients in the herbs are much more easily absorbed through the moist lining of the digestive tract. Most herbs in this book are available as remedies you can easily buy over the counter or obtain by mail order or online, and there is a great deal of variety in different products from different manufacturers. Always read and follow the stated dosage advice, and do not exceed it.

Simple, external methods of use—such as facial steams, baths, macerated oils, compresses, and ointments—have mild effects. Where these are featured in the Directory you will see how often you are recommended to use them. Just follow the instructions.

If you want to use herbs to alleviate a particular problem, such as indigestion, for example, it is best to use just one herb at a time for three to four days, and monitor the results. Too many herbs at once can confuse the system. Always, if symptoms do not improve, seek a physician's or professional herbalist's advice.

SAFETY INFORMATION

Within the Directory, if it is specified that an herb or preparation should be "taken as directed," follow the instructions on the label or packaging in which the product was supplied. If you are in any doubt, consult a professional herbalist for advice.

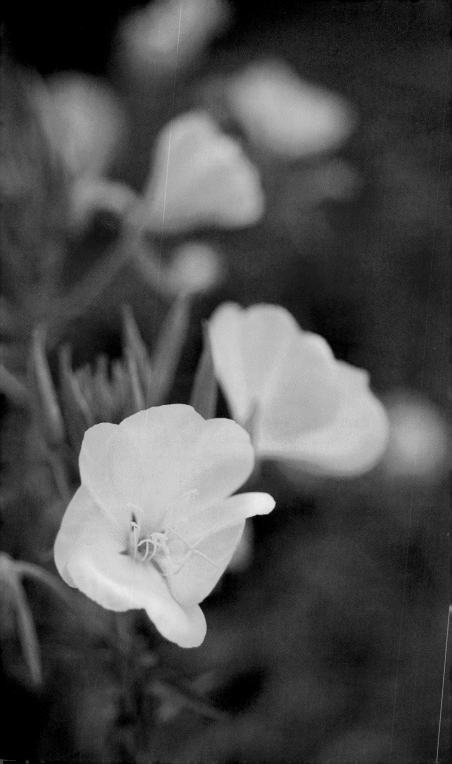

THE HERB DIRECTORY

This section contains 130 individual herb profiles, arranged alphabetically by their botanical Latin names. If you only know an herb by its common name, use the tables on pages 8–11 to find out its botanical name and its location within the Directory.

Each profile provides information on where the herb is native to, what it looks like and where it grows best. Each herb is placed in its historical and cultural context, along with details about its active ingredients and how to use it safely.

If it is specified that an herb or preparation should be "taken as directed," follow the instructions on the label or packaging in which the product was supplied. If you are in any doubt, consult a professional herbalist for advice.

ACHILLEA MILLEFOLIUM
• YARROW

Yarrow is a perennial herb that grows up to 12 in (30 cm) in height, with feathery gray-green leaves and clusters of tiny white and pink flowers that bloom in July, when they are best harvested for drying. It thrives in most soils, in sun or part shade, but it spreads rapidly, thanks to creeping roots and self-seeding, so if you want to feature it in a garden it is best cultivated in a pot to contain it. Other horticultural varieties exist with yellow or bright red flowers but these have no medicinal properties.

In northern Europe yarrow has been valued as a medicinal herb for hundreds of years. The name "yarrow" comes from the Anglo-Saxon term for the plant "gearwe," but it has many descriptive colloquial names in English: "soldier's woundwort," "bloodwort," and "staunchweed" refer to its ability to reduce bleeding and its use as a first-aid herb; "old man's pepper" refers to its use as snuff. In the 17th century the English herbalist Nicholas Culpeper prepared it as an ointment to slow bleeding and shrink hemorrhoids, as well as to heal ulcers or deep wounds. Yarrow flowers, when distilled, yield an essential oil that is bright blue in color, with an anti-inflammatory effect.

SEE ALSO
Peppermint, eucalyptus, comfrey, rosemary

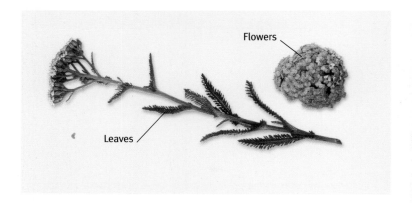

Flowers

Leaves

YARROW

Achillea millefolium

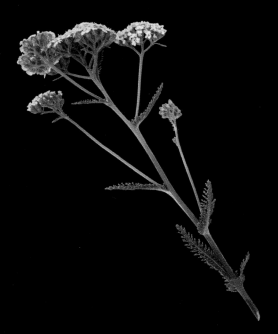

PARTS OF PLANT USED
Flowers, leaves

ACTIVE INGREDIENTS
Alkaloids, amino acid, salicylic acid, saponin, sugar, volatile oil

COMMERCIALLY AVAILABLE AS
Tea, tablets, essential oil

ACTIONS
Analgesic, anti-inflammatory, astringent, diaphoretic

USED TO TREAT
Colds and influenza: an infusion of dried or fresh leaves drunk 2–3 times daily or tablets taken as directed help induce sweating that brings down fevers, especially during viral infections.

Cuts, grazes, wounds: an infusion of fresh or dried leaves (cooled) cleanses injuries and slows bleeding; in an ointment, yarrow encourages the wound-healing process and the formation of new skin cells—apply twice daily.
Rheumatism: in an ointment, yarrow relieves pain and stiffness in joints, as well as backache—massage affected areas gently twice daily. Tablets can also ease pain.

CULINARY USE
None

SAFETY INFORMATION
Prolonged use can lead to headaches and skin sensitivity in sunlight so use for periods of 1–2 weeks only. Avoid in pregnancy—it is a uterine stimulant.

AESCULUS HIPPOCASTUM
• HORSE CHESTNUT

This is a beautiful, majestic-looking tree with wide spreading branches, which grows to well over 100 ft (30 m) in full maturity. It has a smooth grayish-green bark, while the foliage comprises up to five small leaflets with serrated edges joined at a single base. In late spring the tree produces spikes covered with small white flowers with a pink center. In the fall these become sharply spiked shells containing shiny brown nuts. Late October and early November are the best times to collect the nuts for medicinal use. They should be stored in a cool dry place to prevent mold. Horse chestnuts are poisonous to humans when eaten and should not be confused with sweet chestnuts (*Castanea vesca*), which are edible.

Originally horse chestnut trees were native to southeast Europe, and may get their common English name because they have been traditionally used as a protein source for horses and cattle—in countries such as Turkey the nuts were fed to horses to keep them healthy in the winter. Red deer also eat the nuts in the winter to put on a layer of protective fat against the cold. During the 16th century horse chestnut trees were introduced to northern Europe and England, where they naturalized themselves easily.

SEE ALSO
Rosemary, horsetail fern, cayenne pepper, juniper

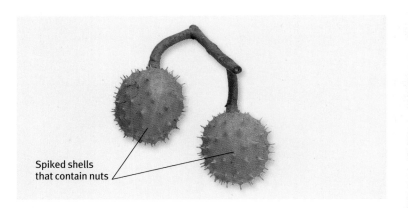

Spiked shells
that contain nuts

HORSE CHESTNUT

Aesculus hippocastum

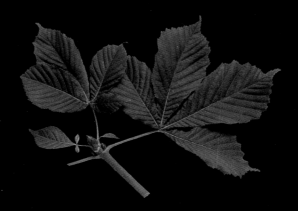

PARTS OF PLANT USED
Ripe nuts, occasionally the bark

ACTIVE INGREDIENTS
Coumarins, flavonoids, glycosides, saponins, tannins

COMMERCIALLY AVAILABLE AS
Ointment, gel, homeopathic tincture

ACTIONS
Astringent, antithrombotic

USED TO TREAT
Varicose veins, aching legs, poor circulation: apply an ointment or gel to varicose veins gently, as directed, to ease pain and assist the circulation to the local area, as well as shrink the veins externally; for tired and aching legs, massage ointment or gel in more deeply twice daily.
Hemorrhoids: apply an ointment or gel to the affected area 2–3 times daily, especially after bowel movements, to soothe pain and itching and encourage shrinkage of swollen veins.

CULINARY USE
None

SAFETY INFORMATION
Homeopathic tincture of horse chestnut should only be used under the guidance of a professional homeopath.

ALCHEMILLA VULGARIS
• LADY'S MANTLE

This perennial herb grows up to 20 in (50 cm) tall with branching hairy stems and velvety leaves with serrated edges. From June to September it also produces masses of tiny yellow flowers. It flourishes in most types of soil, and can be found growing wild in pastures, hedgerows, or woodland areas. If you are planting it in the garden, it likes full sun but will tolerate some shade. The flowers and leaves are best harvested in late June or early July when they are high in active ingredients; they must be dried slowly and stored in the dark to maintain their potency.

The name "Lady's mantle" was first given to the plant in the 16th century by the German botanist Hieronymus Tragus, partly referring to the Virgin Mary ("Our Lady") because of its use to treat female problems, and also because the leaf is shaped like an old-fashioned lady's cloak. The name *Alchemilla* relates to alchemy, a primitive form of chemistry that attempted to manipulate the elements. The surface of the Lady's mantle leaf is covered with tiny hairs where perfect spherical drops of dew form—historically these droplets were collected and consumed because they were believed to have magical powers.

SEE ALSO

Agnus castus, sage, black cohosh, peppermint, lavender

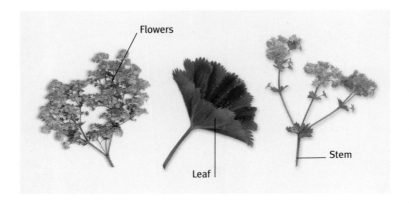

Flowers

Leaf

Stem

LADY'S MANTLE

Alchemilla vulgaris

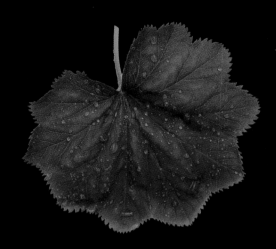

PARTS OF PLANT USED
Flowers, stems, leaves

ACTIVE INGREDIENTS
Bitter compounds, saponins, salicylic acid, tannins, volatile oil

COMMERCIALLY AVAILABLE AS
Tincture, dried capsules

ACTIONS
Anti-inflammatory, antispasmodic, astringent, diuretic, emmenagogue

USED TO TREAT
PMS and menstrual pain: the tincture taken as directed, or an infusion of the leaves drunk twice a day, can relieve painful menstrual cramps and mood swings.

Menstrual and menopausal hormonal imbalance: the tincture or tablets taken as directed ease mood swings, energy fluctuations, and irregular periods.
Diarrhea, digestive cramps, indigestion: the tincture or tablets taken as directed soothe pain and digestive discomfort.
Wounds, damaged skin, insect bites: a strong infusion of the leaves stops bleeding, cleans wounds or cuts, and calms itching bites.
Insomnia: the tincture or capsules taken as directed improve relaxation and sleep.

CULINARY USE
None

SAFETY INFORMATION
Avoid during pregnancy because it stimulates menstruation.

ALLIUM SATIVUM
• GARLIC

This perennial herb produces tall, thin, dark green leaves up to 2 ft (60 cm) high, and purplish white flowers enclosed in papery bracts (enlarged petals). The active part is the bulb that forms below ground, divided into individual "cloves." Cultivation of garlic involves planting cloves in the fall, in rich soil, and a sunny position. The following year, when the plant has flowered and the leaves start to wilt and dry out in the summer, the new bulbs need to be dug up and allowed to dry in the sun before being stored in a cool dry place. They can be used either for culinary or medicinal purposes or for further planting the following season.

Originally native to India and central Asia, garlic is now cultivated all over the world. Horticultural sources suggest it was probably introduced to Britain by the Romans. The Greek writer Herodotus tells that the builders of the Egyptian pyramids ate large quantities of it to give them strength. The name "garlic" derives from Anglo-Saxon "gar" (spear) and "leac" (leek), possibly because the leaves look like those of a leek and the cloves like spearheads.

SEE ALSO
Echinacea, thyme, elder, yarrow, ginger

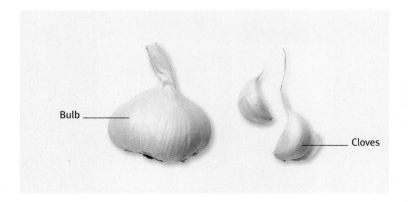

Bulb _____

_____ Cloves

GARLIC
Allium sativum

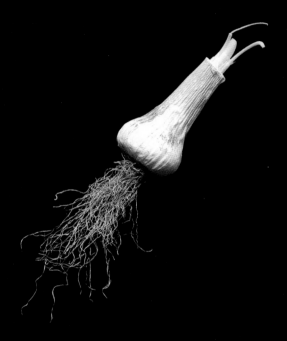

PART OF PLANT USED
Fresh or dried cloves

ACTIVE INGREDIENTS
Diallyl disulphide, which breaks down when the surface is cut to produce the most active ingredient allicin, plus other sulfur compounds; amino acids, fatty oil, vitamins A and C.

COMMERCIALLY AVAILABLE AS
Capsules, tablets, fresh bulb

ACTIONS
Antibacterial, antimicrobial, antiviral, antifungal, anticoagulant

USED TO TREAT
Influenza, viruses, low immunity, respiratory infections: capsules or tablets taken as directed boost the immune system to help fight off infection.
Fungal infections: capsules or tablets taken as directed help increase the efficiency of the immune system to fight yeast infections (candida).
High blood pressure: tablets or capsules taken under medical guidance will help to reduce fatty deposits in the blood and to lower blood pressure.

CULINARY USE
A pungent flavoring in European, Indian, Middle Eastern, and Far Eastern cuisine.

SAFETY INFORMATION
Not to be used medicinally by people taking Warfarin or other anticoagulant medication.

ALOE VERA
• ALOE VERA

This is a succulent plant that grows up to 1–2 ft (30–60 cm) tall, with no stem, producing thick, fleshy leaves that contain a bitter juice and sacs full of gel that oozes out when the leaves are cut. The plants have to be at least three years old before their juice and gel can be collected. In colder, northern climates aloe plants need to be grown in conservatories or greenhouses at a minimum temperature of 41°F (5°C), and in pots with well-drained soil. In their native hot climates they can be grown outside, but they prefer strong sunlight and intense heat. The aloe plant is originally native to East and South Africa.

The aloe plant has been known for its medicinal properties since ancient Greek times. Dioscorides, a famous Greek practitioner of herbal medicine in the 1st century CE used it as a purgative medicinal drug. In northern Europe, references to it occur in 10th-century Anglo-Saxon texts relating to medicinal ingredients; it is presumed to have found its way north via trade routes with Egypt and Africa. In the 17th century aloe vera was successfully introduced to the West Indies where it flourishes to this day and is used in local natural medicine to treat skin complaints.

SEE ALSO
Red clover, camomile, yarrow, lavender, spearmint, cardamom

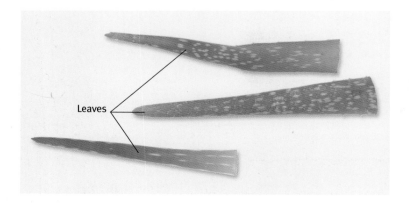

Leaves

ALOE VERA

Aloe vera

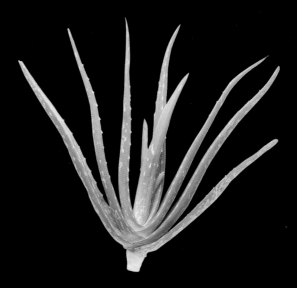

PART OF PLANT USED
Fresh leaves

ACTIVE INGREDIENTS
Juice—glycosides, anthraquinones, resins; gel—anthraquinones, saponins, salicylic acid, vitamins C and E, minerals

COMMERCIALLY AVAILABLE AS
Juice, capsules, tablets, gel

ACTIONS
Anti-inflammatory, digestive tonic, purgative, emollient, wound healer

USED TO TREAT
Eczema, psoriasis, shingles: apply gel to damaged skin areas 2–3 times daily to ease pain, heal open areas, and improve skin regeneration and elasticity.

Burns, cuts, wounds: apply aloe gel 2–3 times daily to clean and disinfect areas, to reduce inflammation, and heal damaged skin.
Indigestion, irritable bowel syndrome, constipation: drink the juice twice daily as directed to improve the health of the bowel and regulate movements.

CULINARY USE
None

SAFETY INFORMATION
Skin application of the gel is safe for all; the juice or capsules should not be taken internally during pregnancy, as aloe can stimulate menstrual flow.

ANEMONE PULSATILLA
• PASQUE FLOWER

A small plant up to 1 ft (30 cm) tall, pasque flower grows from thick, woody roots, producing silky stems covered in silvery white hairs. Its leaves are tiny branching clusters of three segments connected to a single stem, while its flowers are small and violet in color, also covered in hairs. Once it has flowered the plant produces seeds with long feathery tails. For medicinal purposes the plant is harvested at the flowering stage, and then must be dried to destroy a poisonous ingredient called "anemonin." The dried plant deteriorates quickly and must be used within a year.

The name "pasque flower" refers to the feast of Easter, this being a spring flowering plant. The juice of the exterior flower petals yields a green dye; in the past, people in many European countries used it to create decorative patterns on hardboiled eggs—the original "Easter eggs." The ancient Greek herbal practitioner Dioscorides used the flower to make a remedy for eye problems, and it is interesting to note that modern homeopathy uses this plant to make a remedy known as "pulsatilla" to help tearfulness.

SEE ALSO
Black cohosh, agnus castus, clary sage, saw palmetto

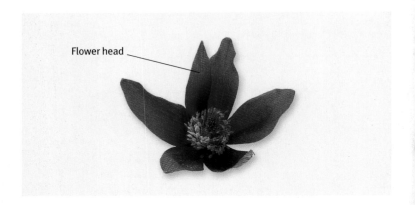

Flower head

PASQUE FLOWER

Anemone pulsatilla

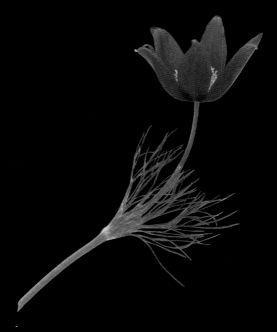

33

PART OF PLANT USED
Dried flowering tops

ACTIVE INGREDIENTS
Glycosides, resin, saponins

COMMERCIALLY AVAILABLE AS
Capsules, tablets, homeopathic pills
and tincture

ACTIONS
Nervous restorative, antispasmodic,
analgesic

USED TO TREAT
*Headache, migraine, PMS, nervous
exhaustion:* capsules, tablets or
homeopathic preparations can be taken
as directed to relieve headaches or
mood-related menstrual symptoms.

Menstrual pain and cramps: capsules
or tablets can be taken as directed to
relieve pain and menstrual discomfort.
Male reproductive dysfunction: capsules,
tablets or homeopathic preparations can
be taken as directed to relieve stress-
related sexual difficulties.

CULINARY USE
None

SAFETY INFORMATION
The fresh plant is poisonous due to
an ingredient called anemonin, which
is destroyed during drying. This is a
powerful herb and should only be taken
in its dried form under the guidance of
a professional herbal practitioner. The
homeopathic remedy is safer for use as
an emotional and anxiety support.

ANETHUM GRAVEOLENS
• DILL

Dill is a member of the same plant family as cilantro, angelica, and fennel, closely resembling the latter except that it is an annual and shorter at only 3 ft (1 m) tall. It has a single straight stem and many aromatic wispy leaves, and produces "umbels"—umbrella-shaped clusters of tiny yellow flowers that become flat oval seeds. Originally native to the Mediterranean it is now cultivated all over the world. Seeds should be sown in late spring in well-drained, nutrient-rich soil, and watered daily. Dill is best planted away from fennel to avoid cross-pollination. The leaves can be eaten fresh or used to make infusions. The seeds should be harvested in late summer—cut the flower heads and hang them upside down with a paper bag tied around them securely (the seeds will fall into the bag).

34 As far back as the 1st century CE, the Greek herbal expert Dioscorides described a plant he called "anethon," which is believed to have been dill. It has been used as a digestive remedy since early medieval times. The name is derived from the Norse "*dilla*" (meaning "to calm"), and refers to the plant's soothing properties. In the 17th century the English herbalist Nicholas Culpeper used the seeds to strengthen the mind and dispel depression.

SEE ALSO
Fennel, chervil, peppermint, ginger, cilantro

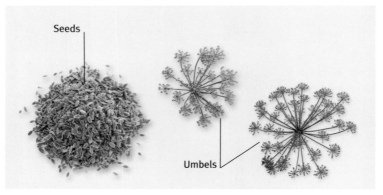

Seeds

Umbels

DILL

Anethum graveolens

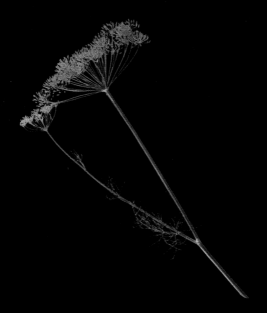

PARTS OF PLANT USED
Fresh leaves, seeds

ACTIVE INGREDIENTS
Particularly in the seeds—fatty oil, mucilage, tannins, volatile oil

COMMERCIALLY AVAILABLE AS
Gripe water, herb tea, fresh herb

ACTIONS
Digestive tonic, antispasmodic, sedative

USED TO TREAT
Indigestion, stomach cramps: an infusion of fresh dill leaves relieves gas and eases painful digestive trouble; herbal gripe water containing dill seed is available commercially and is good for children aged five or over.

Constipation, Irritable Bowel Syndrome (IBS): to help soothe cramps and regulate bowel rhythm, grind up one teaspoon of dill seeds and make into an infusion.

CULINARY USE
Fresh leaves add a subtle aniseed taste to fish dishes, soups, cucumber, cheese and egg recipes; the seeds are used in chutneys and pickles.

SAFETY INFORMATION
No issues

ANGELICA ARCHANGELICA

• ANGELICA

Angelica is a dramatic-looking aromatic plant that grows to 4–8 ft (1.2–2.4 m) in height, and has hollow stems, large, pale green leaves and globular umbels of yellow-green flowers, followed by flat seeds. It needs moist, rich soil and full sun, and can be sown from ripe seeds, which should be planted in August or propagated by dividing roots. To harvest roots for medicinal purposes, dig up a section in the fall of the first year; wash it and leave it to dry in a linen closet, then store in an airtight jar. Herbal suppliers sell dried angelica root chopped into small pieces for use as a medicinal remedy.

For hundreds of years angelica has been revered as a blood purifying and anti-infectious herb. Biblically it has been associated with the protective archangels Michael and Gabriel, and during the Great Plague in the 17th century the roots were chewed to protect against infection. Today it is used in western herbal medicine as a cleansing and detoxifying remedy. Essential oil of angelica root is also used in professional aromatherapy treatments as an ingredient in massage blends to combat cellulite.

SEE ALSO

Dill, fennel, cilantro, peppermint, yarrow, cayenne pepper

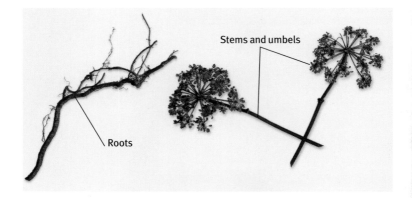

Stems and umbels

Roots

ANGELICA

Angelica archangelica

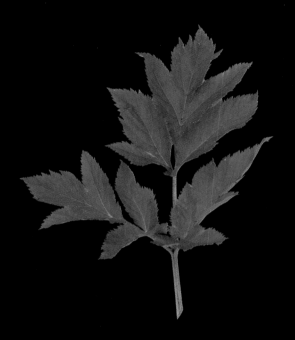

PARTS OF PLANT USED
Roots, seeds

ACTIVE INGREDIENTS
Bitters, glycosides, organic acids, sugar,
tannins, volatile oil

COMMERCIALLY AVAILABLE AS
Dried root, essential oil, herbal teas,
tincture

ACTIONS
Digestive tonic, antispasmodic,
expectorant

USED TO TREAT
Coughs and bronchitis: an infusion
of dried root taken 2–3 times daily
eases the irritation that causes
spasmodic coughs.

Indigestion, cramps: an infusion of dried
root or tincture taken as directed calms
digestive cramps and helps the liver to
digest fatty or rich foods.
Rheumatic pain: 1 tablespoon of
dried root in a small muslin bag added
to a hot bathtub eases pain and
improves circulation.

CULINARY USE
Young angelica stems boiled in sugar
are used as candied fruit in baking;
seeds and root are used to make
liqueurs such as Benedictine.

SAFETY INFORMATION
Angelica root, seed or essential oil may
cause photosensitivity. All forms of
angelica should be avoided in pregnancy
as they can cause uterine contractions.

ANGELICA SINENSIS
• DONG QUAI

This perennial aromatic herb is one of the vast botanical family *Apiaceae* that includes fennel, cilantro, carrot, celery, angelica, and dill. It is native to Japan and China and thrives in cold, damp, mountainous regions. Dong quai can grow up to 8 ft (2.4 m) tall, with light green leaves divided into smaller leaflets and flat umbrella-like clusters ("umbels") of white flowers. Its yellow-brown roots are the medicinal component; they are thick and woody, containing several important and powerful ingredients. Harvesting involves digging them up, washing them and drying them to preserve their potency.

The common name "dong quai" is an anglicized spelling of the Chinese name, sometimes written as "dang gui" or "tang kui." Its other common name is Chinese angelica. It has been used for hundreds of years in traditional Chinese medicine as a so-called "female ginseng," to treat menstrual, menopausal, and hormonal problems in women, as well as anemia and high blood pressure. It is a powerful herb with a strong tonic effect on the feminine reproductive system; its regular use should be discussed with a professional medical herbalist.

SEE ALSO

Black cohosh, sage, agnus castus, clary sage, Lady's mantle

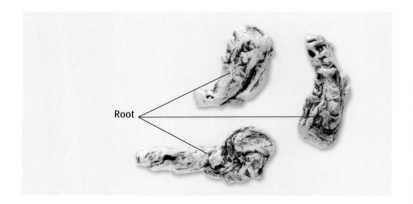

Root

DONG QUAI

Angelica sinensis

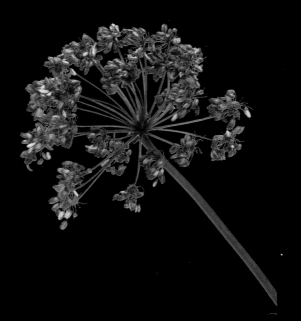

PART OF PLANT USED
Root

ACTIVE INGREDIENTS
Flavonoids, minerals, phytosterols, vitamins, volatile oil

COMMERCIALLY AVAILABLE AS
Ointment, capsules, tincture

ACTIONS
Antispasmodic, hormone regulating, uterine tonic, analgesic, anti-inflammatory, sedative

USED TO TREAT
Menstrual cramps, irregular menstruation, hormone imbalance: tablets or tincture taken as directed ease spasms and regulate menstrual flow.

Menopausal symptoms: tablets or tincture taken as directed compensate for falling estrogen levels, alleviating symptoms such as hot flashes.
High blood pressure: tablets or tincture taken as directed under medical guidance help to reduce blood pressure and decrease fatty deposits.

CULINARY USE
None

SAFETY INFORMATION
Avoid during pregnancy. Can increase skin sensitivity to UV light. Should not be taken by women with a history of breast, ovarian, or uterine cancer, or by men with a history of prostate cancer. It should be avoided by anyone taking anticoagulant medication such as Warfarin.

ANTHEMIS NOBILIS
• ROMAN CAMOMILE

Roman camomile is related to German camomile (*Matricaria chamomilla*, pages 164–5); however it has a milder effect and more pleasant aroma. It is a perennial herb growing to 1 ft (30 cm) in height, with feathery, aromatic leaves and pale yellow flowers. The whole plant has a strong apple-like aroma, and it is a very useful plant to grow in a garden because it attracts insects that prey on pests such as greenfly. A particular horticultural variety of Roman camomile known as "treneague" does not produce flowers; this can be planted as a lawn that releases its aroma as you walk on it. Roman camomile flowers are important medicinally; they need to be picked in summer at full bloom and then carefully dried before use.

The name "camomile" comes from the Greek "*khamai melon*," which literally means "earth apple." This is a good description, because the herb is low-growing and smells strongly of apples. A classic sedative herb throughout the history of western herbal medicine, today Roman camomile is often combined with similar-acting herbs and made into tablets to help promote natural sleep. Essential oil of Roman camomile is commonly used in aromatherapy to help skin problems and insomnia.

SEE ALSO
Lavender, red clover, St. John's wort, German camomile, valerian

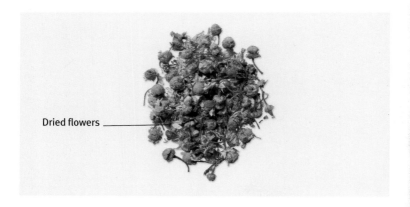

Dried flowers

ROMAN CAMOMILE

Anthemis nobilis

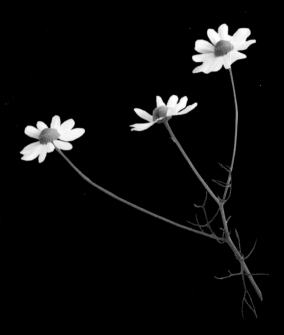

PART OF PLANT USED
Flowers

ACTIVE INGREDIENTS
Bitter compounds, glycosides, volatile oil

COMMERCIALLY AVAILABLE AS
Dried flowers, teas, tablets, tincture, essential oil

ACTIONS
Analgesic, anti-inflammatory, antispasmodic, sedative

USED TO TREAT
Insomnia due to stress, anxiety, mood swings: herbal tea drunk twice daily or capsules taken as directed or three drops of essential oil in a warm bathtub will enhance relaxation and ease emotional stress.
Indigestion, nausea: 3 drops of essential oil in 1 teaspoon of sunflower oil massaged into the abdomen twice daily eases indigestion; herbal tea drunk twice daily will do the same.
Skin irritation, eczema, nettlerash (hives), burns, sunburn: infusion of dried flowers, cooled and applied to skin, soothes irritation and calms redness or itching; 3 drops of essential oil in 1 teaspoon of sunflower oil applied to an area calms redness and speeds healing.

CULINARY USE
None

SAFETY INFORMATION
No issues

ANTHRISCUS CEREFOLIUM
• CHERVIL

Chervil is a hardy annual plant 1–2ft (30–60cm) tall, with bright green feathery leaves and flat umbels of tiny white flowers in early summer. This herb can be found in the wild but there are several poisonous species that resemble it, so it is best to buy seeds from a reputable supplier and grow your own. It prefers light, moist soil, and a sunny location, and is easily grown from seed in early spring, in the garden, in pots, or on a windowsill. For culinary purposes, as the plant matures, cut away any flowering stalks—this makes it produce more useful aromatic leaves. Chervil is a lovely herb to choose for a culinary collection in pots or in a small herb plot, with other useful companions such as parsley, tarragon, chives, rosemary, and thyme.

In medieval Europe, chervil was valued as a useful medicinal remedy to cleanse the kidneys and liver. It was also used to bathe the eyes. The 17th century English herbalist Nicholas Culpeper regarded it as a warming remedy to ease troublesome indigestion and menstrual cramps. It is not popular in herbal medicine today, but included in the diet it has beneficial effects on the digestive system.

SEE ALSO
Fennel, cilantro, mustard seed, tarragon, black pepper

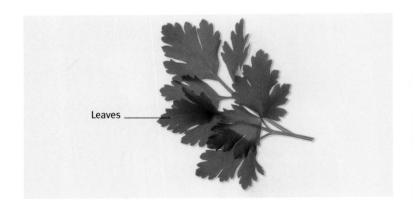

Leaves ———

CHERVIL

Anthriscus cerefolium

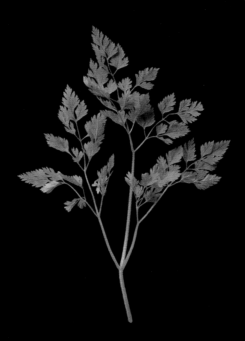

PART OF PLANT USED
Fresh leaves

ACTIVE INGREDIENTS
Volatile oil

COMMERCIALLY AVAILABLE AS
Fresh or dried culinary herb

ACTIONS
Digestive cleanser and liver tonic

USED TO TREAT
Chervil was used medicinally in the past but today it does not feature in herbal medicine. It is an example of an aromatic plant with digestive tonic benefits that are best experienced through the diet.

CULINARY USE
Fresh chervil leaves are used extensively in French cooking; they add a delicate aniseed flavor to butters, soups, sauces, salad dressings, and taste very good in omelettes and egg dishes or with chicken. They need to be added at the end of cooking or as a garnish as the flavor and beneficial dietary effect is lost through overheating. Flat-leaved French parsley works well in combination with chervil as an aromatic and digestive tonic-herb combination.

SAFETY INFORMATION
No issues

APIUM GRAVEOLENS

• CELERY SEED

Celery is well known as a vegetable, with its clean, fresh, tangy taste, and is one of the three most popular salad ingredients in the world. The crunchy stalks are called "petioles," meaning they are special thickened leaves. Sprouting upper leaves are cut off on commercially bought celery, but if the bulb is left in the ground, the upper leaves eventually branch into dark green umbels of pale yellow flowers, which produce pungent aromatic seeds. The species of celery we commonly eat was originally native to the Mediterranean region; however, various related wild species are found in the British Isles, Sweden, Middle Eastern countries such as Egypt, parts of the United States, South America, and China.

The Romans were the first to eat celery as a vegetable, and the Italians began cultivating it domestically in the 17th century, eliminating its more bitter flavors and producing thicker, tastier leaves. They also developed the technique of blanching, meaning piling soil around the stalks to keep them pale and milder flavored. In Ayurveda—the ancient traditional medicine of India—celery seeds are a staple remedy, and are still used today to treat conditions including indigestion, water retention, arthritis, and poor liver function.

SEE ALSO
Fennel, grapefruit, lemon, dandelion, cranberry

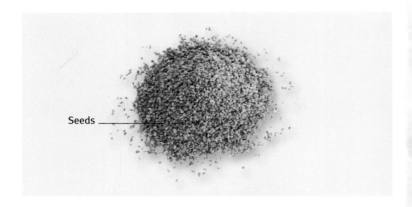

Seeds

CELERY SEED
Apium graveolens

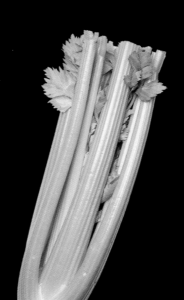

PART OF PLANT USED
Seeds

ACTIVE INGREDIENTS
Volatile oil

COMMERCIALLY AVAILABLE AS
Capsules, tincture

ACTIONS
Diuretic, carminative, liver tonic, antirheumatic, anti-inflammatory

USED TO TREAT
Water retention, bloating: tablets or tincture taken as directed will stimulate urinary flow and encourage detoxification.
Indigestion, stomach cramps, gas: tablets or tincture taken as directed relieve painful spasms and excess gas in the bowel.
Gout, osteoarthritis, rheumatism: Tablets or tincture taken as directed help to encourage the excretion of uric acid, which forms crystalline deposits around the joints in gout or arthritis; celery seed extract relieves inflammation and pain.

CULINARY USE
None

SAFETY INFORMATION
Celery seed extract should not be taken during pregnancy because of the strong diuretic effect. Prolonged oral doses may cause skin sensitivity to UV light. Because of the strong diuretic effect, be sure to replace lost fluid with pure spring water to avoid dehydration.

ARCTIUM LAPPA
• BURDOCK

A biennial plant eventually growing to a height of 3–4 ft (1–1.2 m), burdock produces a rosette of large, heart-shaped leaves in the first year of growth, and in the second year a tall stem with smaller leaves covered with soft, downy hairs. The flowers are produced in late summer and early fall; they have purple crowns on top of thistle-like clusters of prickles commonly known as "burrs," hence the name of the plant. Native to northern Europe, burdock is still a prolific wild plant, found growing in profusion in light, well-drained soil on waste ground or in hedgerows. It can be easily cultivated from seed. For medicinal purposes the root from one-year-old plants is the most potent, harvested in July and dried.

William Shakespeare, an astute observer of plants, included references to many common flowers and herbs in his plays: in *Troilus and Cressida* the character Pandarus says, "They are burs, I can tell you, they'll stick where they are thrown," an allusion to the clusters of prickles that cling very efficiently to clothing. Nicholas Culpeper, the 17th-century English herbalist, used the roots to help constipation, infectious fevers and kidney stones. Although the root is most commonly used in herbal medicine today, in the past the leaves were used to calm indigestion and the seeds to soften the skin.

SEE ALSO
Tea tree, yarrow, black pepper, ginger, cardamom

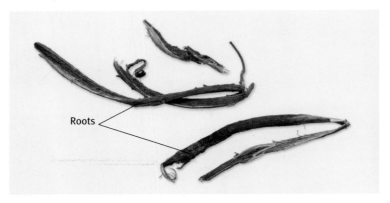

Roots

BURDOCK
Arctium lappa

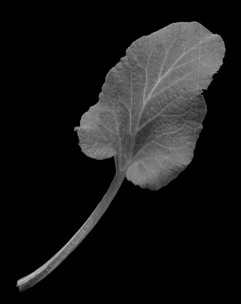

PART OF PLANT USED
Roots

ACTIVE INGREDIENTS
Mucilage, resin, starch, tannins, volatile oil

COMMERCIALLY AVAILABLE AS
Capsules, tablets, tincture

ACTIONS
Diuretic, antiseptic, diaphoretic

USED TO TREAT
Influenza, fevers: tablets or tincture taken as directed induce sweating to cool the body and help fight viruses. *Gout, rheumatism:* tablets or tincture taken as directed help rid the body of excess uric acid and other toxins.

Wounds, ulcers, eczema: a decoction of the root boiled in water and cooled will soothe, cleanse, and disinfect areas of damaged skin.

CULINARY USE
None

SAFETY INFORMATION
Safe at recommended levels, do not exceed suggested amount; burdock is best used at lower doses over a longer period of time because its internal cleansing effects can be powerful.

ARCTOSTAPHYLOS UVA-URSI
• BEARBERRY/UVA URSI

A low-growing evergreen shrub with long branches that form a dense mat of foliage, bearberry is a member of the same plant family (*Ericaceae*) as heather (*Erica vulgaris* pages 104–5). The shrub produces small, oval, leathery, dark green leaves and small white flowers. The berries are small, red and shiny, each with five seeds inside. Bearberry thrives in acidic soils on moors, hillsides and in mountainous regions. As a wild shrub it is still found in Scotland and many parts of northern Europe, though it is becoming increasingly rare, and some countries have designated it a protected species. It is commercially cultivated for the leaves, used to make a variety of herbal tablet combinations for urinary and kidney-related complaints. They are collected in September or October when the foliage is most dense, and carefully dried to make herbal preparations.

The botanical name is amusingly descriptive: "arctostaphylos" is from two Greek words, "*arktos*" meaning "bear" and "*staphyle*" meaning "grape;" "*uva*" is the Latin world for "grape" and "*ursi*" is the Latin for "of the bear." Both of these phrases refer to the belief in folklore that bears enjoy the taste of the fruit. The earliest historical references to the plant occur in 13th-century medical documents from Wales, and it has been in continuous use ever since.

SEE ALSO
Celery seed, fennel, juniper, grapefruit, angelica

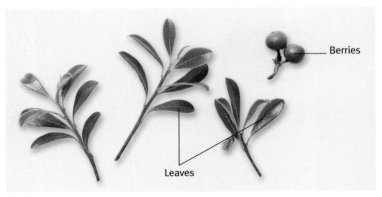

Berries

Leaves

BEARBERRY/UVA URSI

Arctostaphylos uva-ursi

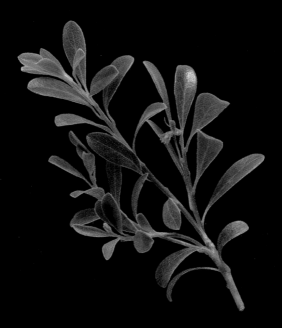

PART OF PLANT USED
Leaves

ACTIVE INGREDIENTS
Glycosides, organic acids, tannins

COMMERCIALLY AVAILABLE AS
Tablets, capsules, tincture

ACTIONS
Diuretic, antiseptic, astringent

USED TO TREAT
Urinary tract infections: tablets, capsules
or tincture taken as directed strengthen
and soothe the urinary tract.
*Fluid retention (including premenstrual),
bloating:* tablets, capsules or tincture
taken as directed stimulate the kidneys
to release excess fluid.

CULINARY USE
None

SAFETY INFORMATION
Do not exceed recommended daily
doses; if you suffer from a medically
diagnosed kidney complaint seek
medical guidance before use.
Long-term use should only be
under the supervision of a qualified
medical herbalist. A vegetarian diet
that keeps the urine alkaline will
improve the efficiency of bearberry's
medicinal actions.

ARMORACIA RUSTICANA
• HORSERADISH

This perennial plant has large, thick leaves that sprout from the base of the stem, and a deep, fleshy taproot containing pungent and powerful medicinal ingredients. Its flowering head is made up of many tiny white blooms, which appear in summer. It prefers moist soil, in which it grows extremely vigorously; once it takes it is very difficult to get rid of. Roots are dug up in the fall for medicinal purposes or to use fresh as a culinary sauce. Young leaves can be picked throughout the season and added to salads.

Both root and leaves have been documented in culinary and medicinal use since the Middle Ages. The plant was popular throughout mainland Europe, renowned for its fiery taste and stimulating effect. In the 16th century the English herbalist John Gerard wrote that horseradish was a strong relish to accompany meat. In 1640 another English herbalist, John Parkinson, described it as a "strong-tasting sauce enjoyed by the working classes." By the 18th century it was finally listed in London as a medicinal remedy for circulatory, rheumatic, and digestive problems.

SEE ALSO
Ginger, black pepper, cinnamon, fennel, mustard seed

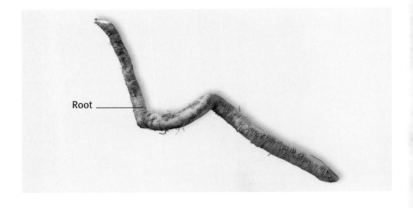

Root

HORSERADISH

Armoracia rusticana

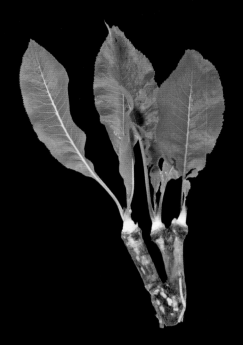

PARTS OF PLANT USED
Roots, leaves

ACTIVE INGREDIENTS
Enzymes, glycosides, resin, vitamin C, volatile oil

COMMERCIALLY AVAILABLE AS
Tincture, tablets

ACTIONS
Strong digestive stimulant, expectorant, circulatory stimulant

USED TO TREAT
Coughs, catarrh, chest congestion: herbal tablets taken as directed help to dry up the mucus deposits that cause chest congestion, and also loosen tight coughs.

Indigestion, especially after red meats and oily food: herbal tablets or tincture taken as directed assist the liver in breaking down heavy fatty ingredients. *Rheumatism, osteoarthritis:* tablets taken as directed help to ease stiff joints and improve local circulation.

CULINARY USE
In Britain horseradish sauce is traditionally eaten with roast beef. Pungent young horseradish leaves can be added to green salads.

SAFETY INFORMATION
Do not use externally on sensitive or allergy-prone skin. Do not eat the root or take as a herbal remedy if suffering from stomach ulcers. Avoid if you have low thyroid function or are taking thyroxine.

ARNICA MONTANA
• ARNICA

This perennial herb, also known as "mountain tobacco," grows up to 1–2 ft (30–60 cm) tall, with a rosette of lance-shaped, pale yellow-green leaves at the base of the stalk, and two or three flower heads per plant, producing a deep golden-yellow daisy-like bloom. Arnica is a member of the vast plant family *Compositae*, which includes calendula, (see pages 66–7), Roman camomile (see pages 40–1), German camomile (see pages 164–5), daisy (see pages 58–9), and sunflower (see pages 134–5). Arnica thrives in hilly or mountainous regions both in Europe and the United States; however, it is often classified as a protected plant in the wild. Both the flowers and the root have medicinal properties, and in early North American herbal practice the blooms were used for pain relief.

Arnica is an example of an herb that is now used differently from former times, because in its natural state it is extremely powerful with an irritant effect if taken internally or applied to the skin. It is most commonly known today as a homeopathic remedy. Homeopathy is able to make use of powerful and sometimes poisonous substances by diluting them many times, to the point where they are hardly present any more. Homeopathic arnica is very safe and effective to use, and is extremely useful as a first-aid remedy.

SEE ALSO
German camomile, yarrow, Roman camomile, lavender, melissa

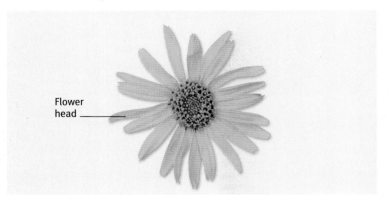

Flower head ————

ARNICA

Arnica montana

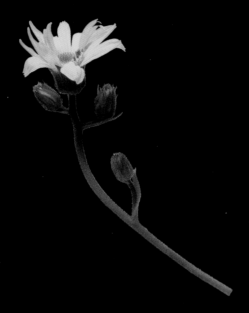

PART OF PLANT USED
Flowers

ACTIVE INGREDIENTS
Bitters, flavonoids, glycosides, saponins, volatile oil

COMMERCIALLY AVAILABLE AS
Homeopathic tincture, cream and ointment, pills

ACTIONS
Anti-inflammatory, analgesic

USED TO TREAT
Bruises, blows and minor injuries: immediate application of arnica cream or ointment to an injury (skin must be unbroken), plus oral dosage of arnica homeopathic pills as directed will stop swelling, reduce bruising, and ease pain.
Shock, hysteria, sudden upset: homeopathic pills or tincture taken as directed help to calm emotional shock and panic.

CULINARY USE
None

SAFETY INFORMATION
The herb arnica is not suitable for external or internal use because of its powerfully irritant effects; however, homeopathic arnica is completely safe to use, even on babies and small children.

ARTEMISIA DRACUNCULUS
• TARRAGON

A perennial herb that grows up to 3 ft (1 m) tall, tarragon has branching stems and narrow, pointed, very aromatic dark green leaves. It produces pale green flowers but only runs to seed in its native hot Mediterranean environment. In cooler areas it has to be propagated by taking cuttings from new spring growth, or by dividing clumps of roots and replanting them separately. It thrives in moist but well-drained soil, and needs full sun. The stems are best harvested just before the flowers bloom, on a dry day. Hang upside down to dry, then gently pull the leaves off the twigs and store in an airtight jar.

The name "tarragon" comes from the French name "*estragon*" or "*herbe au Dragon*," which means "dragon's herb." This may be because the roots look rather like coiled snakes, or because in medieval times tarragon was widely believed to be a cure for insect and snake bites and effective against poisons. It first appeared in English gardens during the 15th and 16th centuries. In the 17th century the English herbalist John Evelyn recommended its use in salads, while Nicholas Culpeper used it as a menstrual tonic.

SEE ALSO
Peppermint, spearmint, fennel, tea tree, garlic

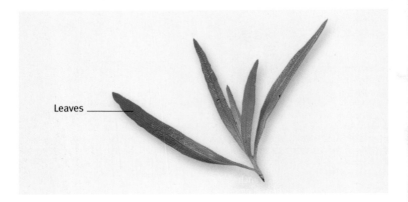

Leaves _____

TARRAGON

Artemisia dracunculus

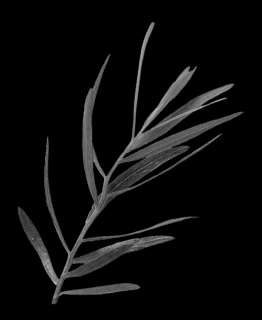

PART OF PLANT USED
Leaves

ACTIVE INGREDIENTS
Bitters, tannins, volatile oil

COMMERCIALLY AVAILABLE AS
Fresh or dried culinary herb, essential oil

ACTIONS
Internally cleansing, liver tonic

USED TO TREAT
Sore gums, mouth ulcers, toothache:
infusion of the fresh leaves, cooled,
disinfects, soothes, and eases pain.

CULINARY USE
Tarragon is a classic herb in French
cuisine, mainly used in cheese, egg, fish
and meat dishes, as well as in patés,
salads and dressings, aromatic vinegars,
oils and herb butters; it also adds
interest to plain root vegetables such
as carrots or parsnips. Because of its
powerful aroma, just three or four fresh
leaves or a pinch of the dried herb are
enough to flavor a dish.

SAFETY INFORMATION
The volatile oil in tarragon leaves is
available as a distilled essential oil
containing an ingredient, estragole,
which is a known abortifacient. The
essential oil and even large doses
of the fresh herb should also be
avoided in pregnancy.

AVENA SATIVA
• OAT

This tall grass grows up to 4 ft (1.2 m) tall, with hollow, jointed stems bearing the flower heads that become the seeds, harvested as oatmeal. Cultivated since ancient Greek times, oats are a vitally important commercial grain crop, now grown all over the world. Ripe oats are harvested in late summer, processed and made available in many grades of oatmeal, from coarse to fine, as well as whole oat flakes. For medicinal purposes and the best digestive effects, try to obtain organically grown oats, guaranteed pesticide-free.

In the 12th century a German abbess and physician called Hildegard of Bingen wrote about the value of oats as a nutrient. She recommended they should be eaten as porridge or oatcakes to rebuild strength and vitality, particularly during periods of physical weakness or illness when the digestion tends to suffer. In the 16th century the English herbalist John Gerard mentions the widespread use of oats in baking throughout northern England, especially as oatcakes, and their use as a staple food in Scotland. In the 17th century, Nicholas Culpeper described how to make a skin wash with oats infused in water to remove freckles from the skin.

SEE ALSO
Lavender, melissa, St John's wort, valerian, passion flower

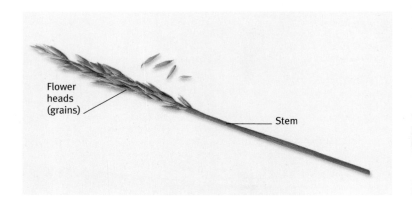

Flower heads (grains)

Stem

OAT

Avena sativa

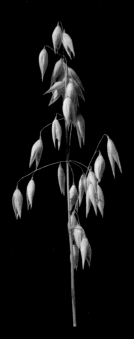

PARTS OF PLANT USED
Oat grains, sometimes stalks

ACTIVE INGREDIENTS
Alkaloids, fat, flavonoids, minerals
(including calcium, copper, iron,
magnesium, silica, and zinc), protein,
saponins (rich source), starch

COMMERCIALLY AVAILABLE AS
Rolled oats, oatmeal, tincture (known as
Avena sativa), tablets

ACTIONS
Internally cleansing, digestive tonic,
nerve restorative, appetite stimulating

USED TO TREAT
Indigestion, recovery after illness: oats
in porridge or soup are nourishing and
easily digested to soothe stomach
discomfort or give energy during recovery.
Dry or sensitive skin: 3 tablespoons
of oats in a small muslin bag added to
a bathtub will soften and soothe the
skin; 2 teaspoons of oats 5 fl oz (150
ml) boiling water, infused then cooled,
soothes sunburn or itching.
*Stress, emotional or nervous tension,
insomnia:* the tincture is a well-known
non-addictive remedy for sleeping
problems and anxiety.

CULINARY USE
In porridge, or baked into oatcakes or
cookies, or added to bread mixtures.

SAFETY INFORMATION
Not recommended for people allergic
to gluten.

BELLIS PERENNIS
• DAISY

This is the humble little white flower with a golden centre that loves to grow in green grass—the common daisy. While perfectionist gardeners would rather eradicate it with weed killer, it might pay to keep it—the flowers have medicinal properties that have been long forgotten. One example is their soothing effect on bruises, which is somewhat similar to arnica (pages 52–3), though much milder. Daisies are perennial, with flowers that open at daybreak and track the sun through changing warmth and daylight—hence the name daisy, from the Old English "day's eye."

In the past, the daisy was valued as an herbal remedy because of its easy availability. As a first-aid treatment for bruises and wounds, or a soothing cough medicine, it played an important part in daily life and was recorded in many old herbal documents as a folk medicine. If you want to use daisies for making herbal preparations such as ointment or macerated oil (see pages 298–9), pick the flowers and use them fresh on the day, as they wilt quickly.

SEE ALSO
Red clover, German camomile, rose, arnica, white horehound

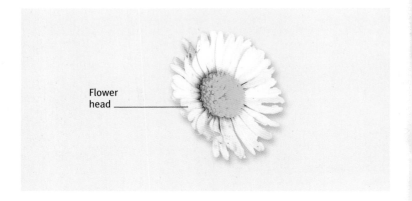

Flower head _____

DAISY

Bellis perennis

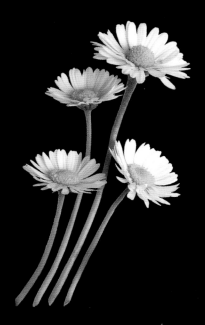

PART OF PLANT USED
Flower heads

ACTIVE INGREDIENTS
Bitters, flavonoids, mucilage, tannins, volatile oil

COMMERCIALLY AVAILABLE AS
Not in commercial preparations

ACTIONS
Astringent, expectorant, vulnerary, anti-inflammatory

USED TO TREAT
Wounds, cuts, grazes: an infusion of fresh flowers, cooled, and applied to injured areas soothes pain, cleanses dirt, and encourages wound healing.
Bruises: a macerated oil or ointment made with fresh daisy flowers (see pages 298–9) applied gently 2–3 times daily soothes pain and inflammation.
Spots, acne: an infusion of fresh flowers, cooled, makes a soothing and antiseptic skin wash.
Coughs: an infusion of fresh flowers with a teaspoon of honey added, taken 2–3 times daily, soothes a tickly cough.
Indigestion, poor liver function: an infusion of the fresh flowers taken 2–3 times daily eases cramps and supports the liver to digest oily foods.

CULINARY USE
Young leaves taste a bit like spinach and can be added to green salads.

SAFETY INFORMATION
No issues

BETULA PENDULA
• SILVER BIRCH

A tall deciduous tree with a smooth, whitish-silver bark and delicate, graceful branches, growing to around 60 ft (20 m) in height. The leaves are oval with a pointed tip and very serrated edges, and are sticky when they are young due to the resin they contain. The tree produces both male and female flowers. Silver birch is native to Europe and Asia, where it grows in woodland, preferring a slightly sandy soil. In spring, birch sap can be tapped and drawn off—it has a sweet taste, and makes a lovely wine. For medicinal purposes the young leaves are also harvested in spring; they are best used fresh, but can be dried for later processing.

Historically, in northern Europe, there were many folk beliefs associated with birch. On the one hand, it was thought to offer protection against evil spirits; on the other hand, birch sticks bound together also formed the original witch's "broomstick." The branches were widely used in thatching, to make roofs for houses, and birch wood or twigs were used to make many household items such as brooms and knife handles.

SEE ALSO
Angelica, fennel, grapefruit, black pepper, ginger

60

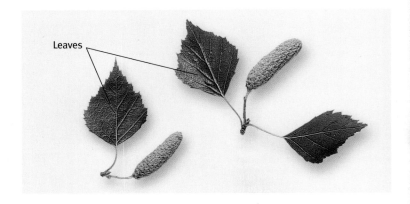

Leaves

SILVER BIRCH
Betula pendula

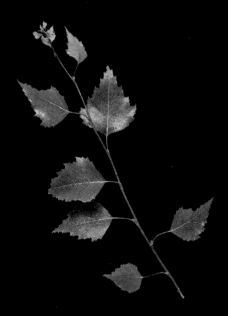

PART OF PLANT USED
Young leaves

ACTIVE INGREDIENTS
Bitters, resin, saponins, tannins, volatile oil

COMMERCIALLY AVAILABLE AS
Teas, tincture, tablets

ACTIONS
Diuretic, disinfectant, diaphoretic, laxative

USED TO TREAT
Bladder and urinary infections: infusion of young leaves drunk 2–3 times daily, or tincture or tablets taken as directed help ease pain and improve the flow of urine.
Rheumatism, arthritis: tincture or tablets taken as directed help ease pain and encourage detoxification via the kidneys.
Poor circulation: a strong infusion of young leaves added to a warm bathtub is an invigorating treatment for cold hands and feet.
Constipation: an infusion of young leaves taken 2–3 times daily acts as a mild laxative to help restore bowel rhythm.

CULINARY USE
None

SAFETY INFORMATION
If you suffer from a medically diagnosed kidney complaint, consult a doctor or medical herbalist before using silver birch. Make sure you drink plenty of fresh spring water to replace lost fluid when using a diuretic remedy.

BORAGO OFFICINALIS
• BORAGE

Borage is a shrub that still grows wild in Britain and parts of Europe, in woodland and on waste ground. It grows 2–3 ft (60–90 cm) tall, and has hollow, hairy stems and pale green, fleshy leaves. It produces bright blue star-shaped flowers from June onward, and is very attractive to bumble bees, being a lovely plant to grow to encourage them into your garden. Sow borage seeds in March in moist but well-drained soil in full sun; once established, plants will then self-seed each year.

The 16th-century herbalist John Gerard said this wild herb made people merry and joyful, driving away all sadness, dullness and melancholy. In the 17th century, Nicholas Culpeper used borage to soothe eye and skin inflammation. Mrs Grieve, a noted 20th-century herbalist, mentions that, because of the pleasant cucumber-like taste and fragrance, young flowering tops of borage can be eaten as early spring greens, and the mature leaves added to salads. Nowadays borage is grown commercially to produce a vegetable oil from its seeds known as "starflower oil," taken as a supplement to balance the skin and hormones.

SEE ALSO
Roman camomile, yarrow, elder, peppermint, evening primrose

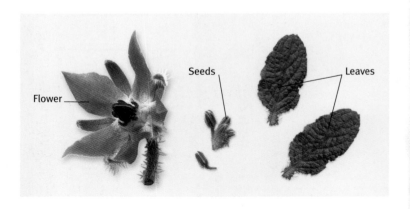

Flower

Seeds

Leaves

BORAGE

Borago officinalis

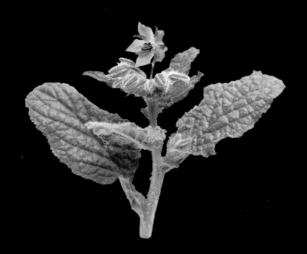

PARTS OF PLANT USED
Flowers, leaves, seeds

ACTIVE INGREDIENTS
High levels of mucilage in the leaves, as well as minerals, saponins, tannins; oil rich in fatty acids in the seeds, high in GLA (gamma-linoleic acid)

COMMERCIALLY AVAILABLE AS
Oil capsules (known as starflower oil); tincture from leaves and flowers

ACTIONS
Leaves—soothing and restorative; seeds (oil)—hormone regulating

USED TO TREAT
Indigestion caused by emotional stress: an infusion of fresh leaves and flowers drunk 2–3 times daily eases anxiety and improves digestive rhythm.
Inflamed or sensitive skin: an infusion of fresh leaves and flowers, cooled, makes a soothing and cleansing skin wash.
Hormone imbalance, PMS, menopausal symptoms: oil capsules taken as directed regulate the menstrual cycle, and ease mood swings or hot flashes.

CULINARY USE
In Britain, blue borage flowers are traditionally added to summer alcoholic punches such as Pimms, or candied to add color to cake decorations. The blue flowers can also be eaten in salads.

SAFETY INFORMATION
No issues

BRASSICA NIGRA
• MUSTARD SEED (BLACK)

This is an annual herb with a slender taproot and an erect, graceful stem, growing up to 3 ft (1 m) tall. It is a member of the large plant family that includes cabbage and broccoli. Black mustard has simple, spear-shaped upper leaves, and the larger lower leaves divide into several pointed sections. Its bright yellow flowers are succeeded by short, narrow pods, each containing 10 or 12 shiny black seeds harvested in the fall. Native to Europe and Asia, the plant can still be found growing wild in ditches, on stream banks or on waste ground.

Black mustard has been cultivated as a spice and medicine for at least 2,000 years. The ancient Greeks believed it to have been discovered by Aesculapius, the "father" of medicine. It is likely that the Romans, great lovers of pungent flavors, especially mustard, brought it to the British Isles where it naturalized itself. It has been used to make a condiment to accompany meat since the Middle Ages. In classic herbals of the 16th, 17th, and 18th centuries it is acclaimed as a hot and drying remedy. One teaspoon of dried mustard powder added to a bowl of hot water to soak the feet is an old fashioned and effective way to stave off colds and influenza, by bringing intense heat into the body.

SEE ALSO
Cayenne pepper, cinnamon, black pepper, cardamom, ginger

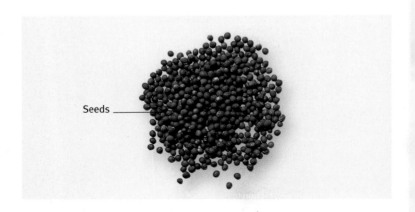

Seeds

MUSTARD SEED (BLACK)

Brassica nigra

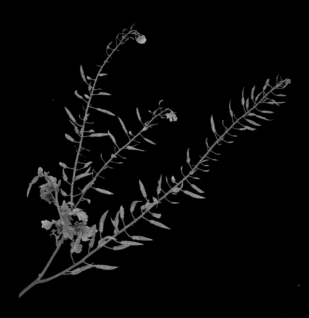

PART OF PLANT USED
Seeds

ACTIVE INGREDIENTS
Alkaloids, enzymes, mucilage, protein, volatile oil

COMMERCIALLY AVAILABLE AS
Dried seeds, massage oil, lotion

ACTIONS
Rubefacient, local circulation stimulant

USED TO TREAT
Muscular aches and pains, pulled muscles, backache: lotion or oil applied to affected area morning and night eases stiffness and pain and improves movement.
Poor circulation: apply oil or lotion to affected areas morning and night with vigorous massage strokes in the direction of the heart to improve circulation.
Rheumatism, arthritis: gently apply oil or lotion morning and night to affected parts, to warm the areas and improve mobility.

CULINARY USE
None

SAFETY INFORMATION
Massage oil or lotion should not be used on individuals with sensitive, allergy-prone skin, or eczema or psoriasis. Always wash hands very thoroughly after application.

CALENDULA OFFICINALIS
• CALENDULA

This attractive annual herb grows up to 20 inches (50 cm) tall, with hairy, slightly sticky leaves. It produces lovely orange flowers, blooming from late spring right through early fall. If you want to grow calendula for medicinal use, plant this exact species—check the botanical name with your seed supplier—because its common name is "marigold" and many horticultural varieties look similar but have no medicinal effects. Calendula is easy to grow in an herb garden, in sunny or part shady spots, and tolerates most soils. Once established, it self-seeds each year. Removing dead flowers ensures a constant supply of new blooms, and flowers should be harvested for drying when they come into full bloom.

The Italians call this herb *"fiore d' ogni mese,"* meaning "flower of every month," because it blooms so regularly. In medieval times it was said that merely looking at the golden flowers strengthened the eyesight, and they were used to make soothing eye washes. Calendula has been used in herbal medicine for hundreds of years to treat fevers, headaches, toothache, and eye and skin problems. It is very simple to make infused calendula oil to help sore, inflamed skin and eczema (see pages 298–9).

SEE ALSO
Lavender, yarrow, aloe vera, fennel, horse chestnut

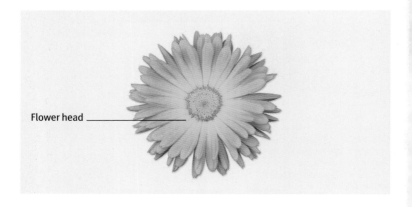

Flower head

CALENDULA

Calendula officinalis

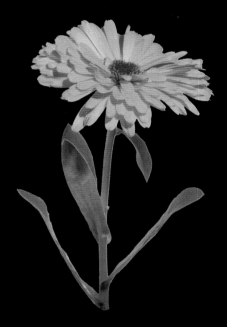

PART OF PLANT USED
Flowers

ACTIVE INGREDIENTS
Bitters, flavonoids, mucilage, resin, volatile oil

COMMERCIALLY AVAILABLE AS
Dried flowers, cream, ointment, massage oil, tincture

ACTIONS
Antiseptic, astringent, bitter, cleansing, diaphoretic, diuretic, vulnerary

USED TO TREAT
Wounds, cuts, inflamed skin: ointment or cream applied 2–3 times daily cleanses damaged areas and encourages skin repair.

Indigestion, poor liver function: drinking infusion of fresh or dried flowers 2–3 times daily improves digestion, especially of fatty foods.
Influenza: infusion of dried or fresh flowers drunk 2–3 times daily helps induce sweating, helping to cool the body and rid it of toxins.
Aching legs, varicose veins: a cream, ointment or massage oil applied twice daily to affected areas with gentle strokes eases aches and itchiness.

CULINARY USE
Fresh petals can be sprinkled on to rice or over salads to add color.

SAFETY INFORMATION
Internal use is not advised during pregnancy due to the hormonal effect.

CAPSICUM FRUTESCENS
• CAYENNE PEPPER

Originally native to South and Central America, India, and Southeast Asia, the cayenne pepper shrub is perennial, growing to 3–6 ft (1–2 m) in height. It has angular branches that are slightly purple at the nodes where they join main stems, and slender leaves. It produces small, long red fruits— chili peppers—containing approximately 20 pungent seeds. Fruit and seeds are harvested and dried for cooking and medicinal purposes. The plant thrives in a tropical climate; in more northern latitudes it needs to be grown in a greenhouse or conservatory, where it may not produce fruit but can make an attractive display in a large pot.

The indigenous races of Central and South America have valued the cayenne for its fiery medicinal properties for hundreds of years. Cayenne appears to have been introduced into Europe in the 16th century; the English herbalist and gardener John Gerard mentioned it in his *General Historie of Plants*, published in 1597, which featured many plants that were new or unusual in his time. In herbal medicine today, cayenne features in many over-the-counter remedies designed to have a warming and stimulating effect on the skin and digestion.

SEE ALSO
Mustard seed, horseradish, ginger, eucalyptus, black pepper

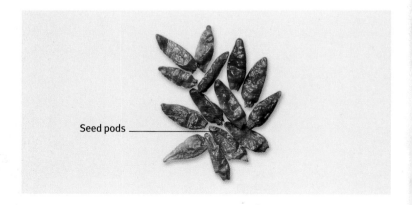

Seed pods

CAYENNE PEPPER

Capsicum frutescens

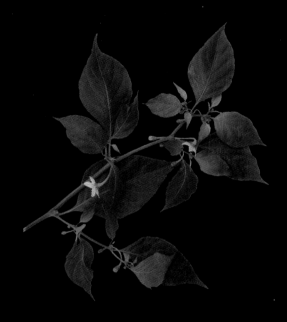

PARTS OF PLANT USED
Pods, seeds

ACTIVE INGREDIENTS
Alkaloid, carotenoids, flavonoids, vitamins, volatile oil

COMMERCIALLY AVAILABLE AS
Dried spice, capsules, tablets, tincture, ointment

ACTIONS
Rubefacient, circulatory stimulant, immune stimulant

USED TO TREAT
Poor circulation, chilblains: ointment applied externally twice daily or tablets, capsules, or tincture taken as directed warm the body and increase blood flow.

Indigestion: tablets or capsules taken as directed warm and stimulate digestive processes in the body.
Muscular aches and pains, pulled muscles, backache: ointment massaged twice daily into affected areas eases pain and improves movement.
Influenza, colds, chills: capsules, tablets, or tincture taken as directed boosts the immune response to viral infections.

CULINARY USE
As chili powder, to season Asian, Mexican, and West Indian recipes.

SAFETY INFORMATION
Use of the ointment is not recommended on broken skin or for those with sensitive allergy-prone skin, eczema, or psoriasis. Wash hands thoroughly after application.

CASSIA ANGUSTIFOLIA
• SENNA

Senna is a North African shrub native to Egypt and Sudan. It grows up to 2 ft (60 cm) tall, has erect, smooth, pale green stems, and long, spreading branches, each bearing around five or seven small grayish-green leaflets. It produces small yellow flowers that mature into pods, each about 2 in (5 cm) long, containing approximately 10 seeds. The seeds, as well as the leaves, are collected twice a year in April and September. The pods and leaves are dried before being processed for medical use. Senna can be grown in cooler climates, but it will rarely flower and will not produce seeds.

Senna has been used medicinally for at least 2,000 years, originally by early Arab physicians ("senna" is an Arabic name). Ancient Greek medical herbalists valued its swift purgative effects that rid the body of excess toxins. The plant's active ingredients include a glycoside called anthroquinone which irritates the lining of the bowel and stimulates internal movement (peristalsis). The effects of senna are fairly immediate, and it is fine to use it occasionally to ease constipation. If irregular bowel rhythm is a constant problem, however, then professional medical advice is needed. Senna is available in a wide variety of commercial herbal preparations, often combined with other digestive tonic herbs to balance its powerful effect.

SEE ALSO
Fennel, celery seed, ginger, mustard seed, slippery elm

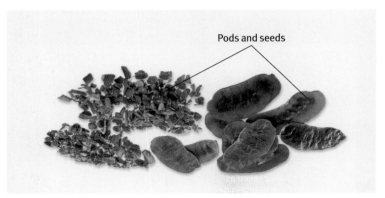

Pods and seeds

SENNA

Cassia angustifolia

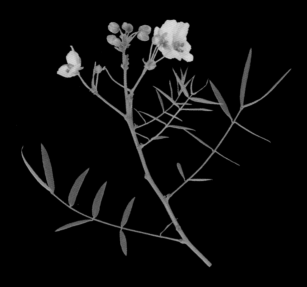

PARTS OF PLANT USED
Leaves, pods, and seeds

ACTIVE INGREDIENTS
Acids, alcohol, glycosides, sugar

COMMERCIALLY AVAILABLE AS
Capsules, tablets, liquid extract, tincture

ACTIONS
Laxative, purgative

USED TO TREAT
Constipation, irregular bowel rhythm:
in tablets senna is usually combined
with fennel or aniseed to prevent
the occurrence of griping pains as it
stimulates the bowel. Tablets, capsules
or liquid extract should be taken as
directed and for no more than 2–3 days;
if symptoms persist, consult a doctor or
medical herbalist.

CULINARY USE
None

SAFETY INFORMATION
Because of the laxative effect, excess
use can lead to vomiting and nausea,
and can impede normal bowel rhythm.
Avoid in pregnancy due to the powerful
stimulating effect. Should not be used
by people with Irritable Bowel Syndrome
(IBS) or colitis, because of the internal
irritant properties of senna.

CENTAUREA CYANUS
• CORNFLOWER

Cornflower is a lovely annual plant growing to 30 in (60 cm) in height, with feathery leaves and tall, tough stems that raise the flowers above the level of ripe corn. Traditionally cornflower grew alongside grain crops in cornfields, before the arrival of pesticides. In the days when corn was reaped by hand, tough cornflower stems were known as "hurt sickle" because they dulled the blades of the sickles used for harvesting. The flowers have daisy-shaped heads with vivid blue petals around a purple center. They can easily be grown from seed straight into the garden in late spring after the last frost, and also do well in pots. Plant them in well-drained soil in full sunlight. Flowers can be picked at full bloom and used fresh or dried for their soothing medicinal properties.

The descriptive botanical name *"Centaurea"* refers to the centaur of Greek myth, the half-man, half-horse called Chiron who taught the healing powers of plants; *"cyanus"* simply means "blue." In the past the flowers were used to make ink, as well as a blue dye for linen.

SEE ALSO
Roman camomile, red clover, eyebright, lavender, oat

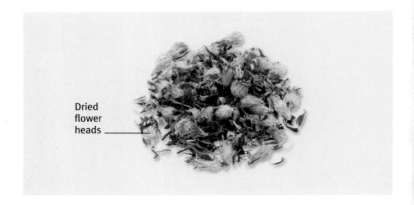

Dried
flower
heads _____

CORNFLOWER

Centaurea cyanus

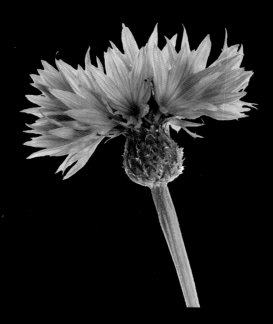

PART OF PLANT USED
Flowers

ACTIVE INGREDIENTS
Blue pigments, mucilage, saponins, tannins

COMMERCIALLY AVAILABLE AS
Tincture

ACTIONS
Diuretic, cleansing, anti-inflammatory

USED TO TREAT
Sore or inflamed eyes, styes: fresh flowers made into an infusion, then cooled, can be applied to the eyes on soaked cotton balls 2–3 times daily. This soothes inflammation, calms itching and heals infection. The commercial tincture can be diluted in water as directed and applied in the same way.
Mouth ulcers: fresh flowers made into a strong infusion, then cooled, can be used twice daily as a mouthwash or gargle with soothing properties. Tincture can also be used as above.
Sensitive or dry skin: fresh flowers made into a strong infusion poured into a warm bathtub is a soothing and calming treatment for sensitive or dry skins.

CULINARY USE
None

SAFETY INFORMATION
No issues, though recurring eye problems or infections should be examined by a doctor or optometrist.

CIMICIFUGA RACEMOSA
• BLACK COHOSH

Black cohosh is a plant from the North American continent, geographically native to Ontario, Georgia, Arkansas, and Wisconsin. It thrives in deciduous forested areas, and is a member of the same family as the buttercup. Above ground it has vibrant green foliage and produces spikes of small, white flowers, blooming from May until September. The knobbly woody root is the active medicinal part, and this was known to many Native American tribes, who gave it names such as "squaw root" because of its beneficial effects on women's health problems.

Black cohosh was also employed by early settlers in the United States to treat menstrual irregularity and to help in childbirth. By the end of the 19th century, the root was given official status by the United States Pharmacopeia. In the early 20th century, research began into the chemistry of black cohosh roots, isolating several active compounds, and in the 1940s the estrogen-enhancing effect was identified. German research from the 1950s has established black cohosh as an effective natural remedy to treat menopausal symptoms. If you are buying black cohosh for this purpose, look for "standardized" supplements guaranteed to contain all its active ingredients.

SEE ALSO
Agnus castus, Lady's mantle, sage, dong quai, borage, evening primrose

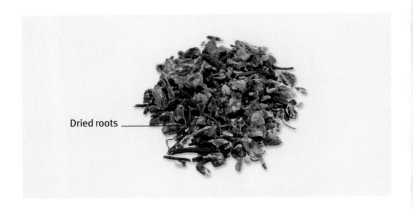

Dried roots

BLACK COHOSH

Cimicifuga racemosa

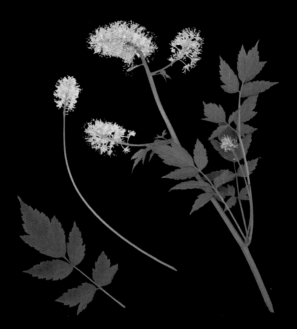

PART OF PLANT USED
Roots

ACTIVE INGREDIENTS
Fatty acids, phytosterols, salicylic acid, sugar, tannins

COMMERCIALLY AVAILABLE AS
Tablets, capsules, tincture

ACTIONS
Estrogen stimulant, sedative, anti-inflammatory

USED TO TREAT
PMS, period pain: capsules, tablets or tincture taken as directed ease menstrual cramps, low energy, and nervous symptoms.
Menopausal symptoms (hot flashes, depression, mood swings): phytosterols in black cohosh have an estrogenic effect, helping to counter many menopausal symptoms, including temperature changes and mood swings.
Headaches, migraine (hormone cycle related): tablets, capsules, or tincture taken as directed help dilute blood vessels in the head and lower blood pressure, easing pain and pressure.

CULINARY USE
None

SAFETY INFORMATION
Excess use can cause stomach irritation and vomiting — do not exceed recommended daily doses. Black cohosh is contraindicated in pregnancy because of the strong hormonal effect.

CINNAMONUM ZEYLANICUM
• CINNAMON

Cinnamon trees are native to hot countries such as Sri Lanka and Malaysia. They grow to 30 ft (9 m) in height, with brown, papery bark, and shiny, tough green leaves. The flowers are creamy white and turn into blue, oval-shaped berries. Cinnamon trees thrive in a tropical climate with plenty of hot sunshine and rain, and a minimum temperature of 59°F (15°C). The commercial spice is made from the dried inner bark of young shoots. Trees are cut back close to the ground to encourage re-sprouting at low level to increase yield when harvesting.

This spice has been a vital medicine, incense and flavoring since Biblical times. In Indian Ayurvedic medicine it is considered an effective remedy for menstrual, respiratory, immune-system, and digestive problems. The world's cinnamon trade was first monopolized by the Portuguese in the 16th century and was then taken over by the Dutch in the 17th century; it was a valuable commodity because of the popularity of the flavor.

SEE ALSO

Peppermint, fennel, spearmint, cardamom, clove, tea tree

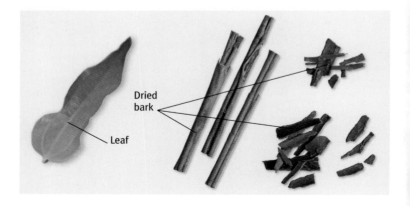

Dried bark

Leaf

CINNAMON

Cinnamonum zeylanicum

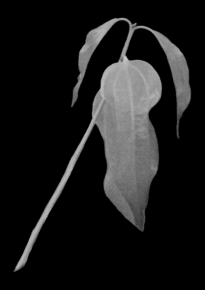

PARTS OF PLANT USED
Inner bark, leaves

ACTIVE INGREDIENTS
Gum, mucilage, tannins, volatile oil

COMMERCIALLY AVAILABLE AS
Whole and powdered spice, tablets, indigestion medicine, essential oil (from leaves)

ACTIONS
Astringent, antifungal, antirheumatic, circulation stimulant, digestive tonic

USED TO TREAT
Indigestion, gas, sluggish digestion: tablets or indigestion formulae taken as directed ease gas in the bowel and stimulate digestive processes.

Colds, influenza, coughs: tablets can be taken as directed to support immune function; cinnamon-leaf essential oil can be used as a soothing inhalation.
Yeast infections (candida): two drops of cinnamon-leaf essential oil added to a warm bathtub soothes irritation.
Rheumatism, osteoarthritis: 2 drops of cinnamon-leaf essential oil added to 2 teaspoons of sunflower oil, massaged into affected areas, improves circulation.

CULINARY USE
As a spice in apple dishes, and in Middle Eastern and Indian savory recipes.

SAFETY INFORMATION
Whole spice is not to be used medicinally during pregnancy. Avoid using essential oil on sensitive skin, or on young children.

CITRUS AURANTIUM
• BITTER ORANGE

The bitter orange tree is evergreen, and grows up to 30 ft (10 m) tall. It has strong leaves with a shiny, dark green upper surface and a paler, matte lower surface. These leaves are pitted with tiny visible glands containing volatile oil, leading to the common French name for the extracted essential oil "*petitgrain*," meaning "little grain." The creamy white flowers of the bitter orange tree have an exquisite fragrance; they are collected and processed to extract one of the most expensive of all essential oils, orange flower, also known as "*neroli*." The tree produces fruit with a very wrinkled peel, used in the making of marmalade. The trees are cultivated for commercial essential oil production in France, Morocco, and Egypt.

Commercial essential oils of orange leaf and flower are easily available (considering the high cost of the flower oil, it is useful to have the leaf oil as a less expensive alternative). The two have fairly similar properties, though the flower oil is used in aromatherapy as one of the best stress-relieving remedies. In southern Mediterranean countries, orange flowers are still a traditional ingredient in bridal bouquets, said to calm wedding nerves.

SEE ALSO
Lavender, oat, valerian, melissa, passion flower

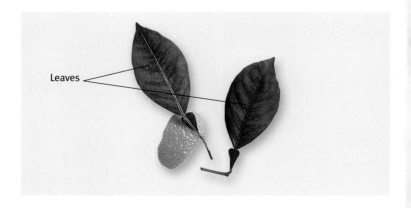

Leaves

BITTER ORANGE
Citrus aurantium

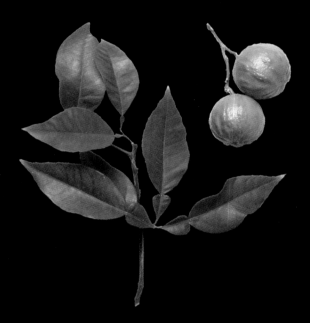

PARTS OF PLANT USED
Leaves, flowers

ACTIVE INGREDIENTS
Volatile oils in leaves and flowers

COMMERCIALLY AVAILABLE AS
Orange-leaf essential oil, orange-flower essential oil (neroli)

ACTIONS
Antispasmodic, cytophylactic, sedative

USED TO TREAT
Oily, combination, or mature skin problems: 2 drops of either leaf or flower essential oil in 1 teaspoon of sunflower oil massaged into the face in the morning and night balances skin oils and improves skin tone.

Indigestion due to stress: 2 drops of either leaf or flower essential oil in 1 teaspoon of sunflower oil massaged clockwise into the abdomen eases stomach cramps.

Insomnia due to stress: 2 drops of leaf or flower essential oil added to a warm evening bathtub enhances relaxation and eases the mind before sleep.

Anxiety attacks: 1 drop of either leaf or flower essential oil on a Kleenex, inhaled, eases panic and worry.

CULINARY USE
Orange-flower water is sometimes used in confectionery.

SAFETY INFORMATION
No issues; the above doses are safe in pregnancy.

CITRUS LIMONUM
• LEMON

Lemon trees are evergreen, and native species have large, sharp thorns protruding from branches. Commercial varieties have been bred to be free of thorns to help with harvesting. Major producing countries today include Brazil, Sicily, and the United States. Lemon leaves are shiny and dark green on the upper surface and paler beneath, pitted with tiny sacs filled with volatile oil. The fragrant flowers are white. Yellow lemon fruit also has visible oil sacs in the peel; pare off a piece of lemon rind and turn it over to see them clearly. When these burst, the zesty lemon aroma is released.

Citrus trees originated in China, and due to early trade routes, cultivation spread into eastern and southern Mediterranean regions in the 14th and 15th centuries, and then to the New World. In the 16th century, eating lemons was encouraged on English ships because this protected sailors from scurvy, a disease caused by lack of vitamin C.

SEE ALSO
Orange, grapefruit, St. John's wort, melissa, lavender

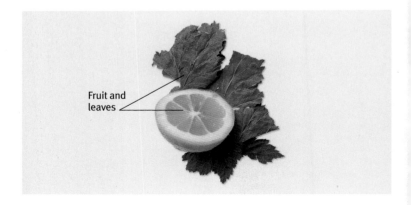

Fruit and leaves

80

LEMON

Citrus limonum

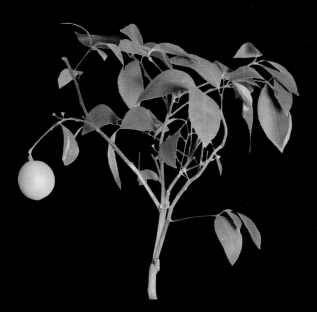

PARTS OF PLANT USED
Peel, leaves

ACTIVE INGREDIENTS
Volatile oils in peel and leaves

COMMERCIALLY AVAILABLE AS
Fruit, essential oils

ACTIONS
Antiseptic, astringent, diuretic,
refreshing aroma

USED TO TREAT
Low immunity, influenza, colds: add 4
drops of lemon essential oil to 1 pint of
boiling water and inhale the steam for 10
minutes as a cleansing inhalation.
Oily and combination skin problems: 2
drops of lemon essential oil added to 1

teaspoon of aloe vera gel massaged into
the face at night clears the pores, heals
spots, and improves skin texture.
Depression, low self-esteem, anxiety:
2 drops of lemon essential oil on a
Kleenex, inhaled, uplifts low moods.

CULINARY USE
Fresh lemon juice is commonly used
with fish dishes, also as a salad dressing
or in baking; lemon peel is a versatile
flavoring in sweet and savory recipes.

SAFETY INFORMATION
Lemon essential oil from the peel used
on the skin can cause irregular patches
of pigmentation in UV light (phototoxity).
Avoid skin use if exposure to sun is
intended. Lemon leaf is safe for skin use
in the sun.

CITRUS X PARADISI
• GRAPEFRUIT

The grapefruit is a hybrid, shown by the "*x*" in the botanical name. It is a cross between the pomelo (*Citrus maximus)* and the sweet orange (*Citrus sinensis*), first grown in Barbados in the 18th century. It is an evergreen tree growing up to 35 ft (12 m) tall, with large, glossy, dark green leaves. It produces highly fragrant creamy-white flowers and the familiar large golden-yellow fruit. The fruit peel is full of sacs containing a volatile oil; if you pare off a thin strip of rind and turn it over, the sacs are clearly visible. When these burst, the bright refreshing aroma of grapefruit is released.

Grapefruit essential oil is pressed or squeezed from the peel. The essential oil is popular in aromatherapy as a refreshing and antidepressant ingredient in massage blends. Grapefruit-seed extract, from the seeds and white flesh, has attracted a lot of publicity in the past 20 years as a possible natural antibiotic and antifungal remedy, but many of these claims have yet to be scientifically proven by clinical trials.

SEE ALSO
Juniper, angelica, celery seed, garlic, myrrh

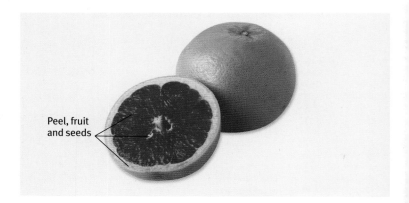

Peel, fruit and seeds

GRAPEFRUIT

Citrus x paradisi

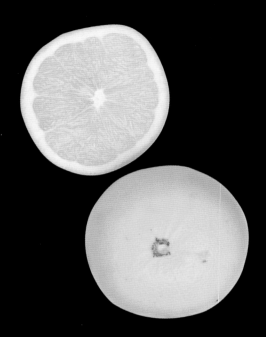

PARTS OF PLANT USED
Peel, seeds

ACTIVE INGREDIENTS
Volatile oil (peel); flavonoids, minerals, sterols, vitamin C (seeds)

COMMERCIALLY AVAILABLE AS
Essential oil (from peel); capsules (seed extract)

ACTIONS
Antiseptic, diuretic, liver tonic, antifungal

USED TO TREAT
Indigestion due to over-rich foods: eating grapefruit, or massaging the abdomen with 2 drops of essential oil in 1 teaspoon of sunflower oil twice daily, calms cramps and improves digestion.

Yeast infections (candida): grapefruit seed extract is said to have antifungal properties; capsules can be taken as directed to help relieve the symptoms of yeast infections.

CULINARY USE
Fresh grapefruit helps detoxify the liver and is reputed to help with slimming.

SAFETY INFORMATION
The essential oil should not be applied to the skin before direct exposure to UV light, because this can cause skin damage (phototoxity). If you are on medication such as Warfarin, eating grapefruit or taking grapefruit-seed extract should be avoided because the drug's effects can be increased. If in doubt check with a doctor.

COMMIPHORA MYRRHA
• MYRRH

This aromatic shrub grows up to 10 ft (3 m) tall, and is very tough, with papery looking, grayish colored bark, and small, oval leaves. The whole shrub is also covered with long, sharp thorns. It bears small white flowers. Whenever its bark is damaged, it produces a reddish resin that dries and crystallizes in contact with heat and air. This seals the bush and protects it from water loss in its natural desert habitat. Myrrh is native to Africa, specifically to Ethiopia and Somalia, and it has been sent along trade routes through Egypt to Europe for thousands of years.

Human beings have been collecting and using myrrh as a wound-healing and antiseptic remedy since antiquity. In the Bible, myrrh is one of the most commonly mentioned aromatic ingredients, along with its botanical relative, frankincense. Myrrh was used in embalming, cosmetic production, wound healing, perfumery, and incense blending from ancient Egyptian times and through the Greek and Roman eras. In the Middle East today, it is still an important ingredient in sacred incense making.

SEE ALSO
Garlic, lemon, tea tree, manuka, clove

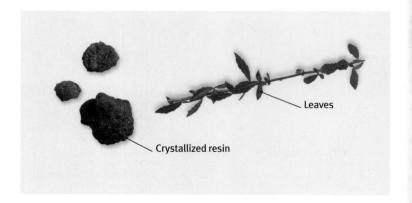

Leaves

Crystallized resin

MYRRH

Commiphora myrrha

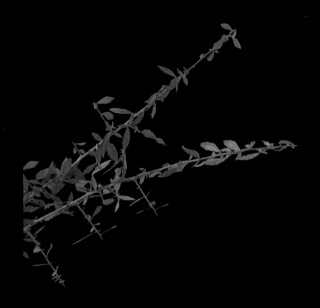

PART OF PLANT USED
Resin

ACTIVE INGREDIENTS
Gum, resins, volatile oil

COMMERCIALLY AVAILABLE AS
Essential oil, gargle/mouthwash, cough syrup, resin, salve, tincture

ACTIONS
Antifungal, antiseptic, astringent, expectorant, vulnerary

USED TO TREAT
Sore gums, mouth ulcers or minor infections: commercial gargle/mouthwash or tincture can be used as directed to soothe inflammation and kill infection.

Yeast infections: commercial gargle/mouthwash can be used as directed to fight oral yeast infections; 2 drops of essential oil can be added to a warm bathtub for vaginal yeast infections.
Athlete's foot: 2 drops of essential oil added to a bowl of warm water and a teaspoon of salt is an effective antifungal foot soak treatment. Repeat twice daily.
Wounds, deep cuts, boils, infected skin: salve can be applied 2–3 times daily to clear infection and increase healing.
Chesty coughs: cough syrup taken as directed eases spasms and breathing.

CULINARY USE
None

SAFETY INFORMATION
Do not use during pregnancy.

CORIANDRUM SATIVUM
• CILANTRO

This annual herb is originally native to the eastern Mediterranean region. It grows up to 2 ft (60 cm) tall, with pungent, divided, feathery leaves, and flat umbels of pale pink and white flowers that become ridged seeds. It is easy to grow from seed; plant it straight out into the garden in late spring after the last frost. Cilantro prefers fertile, well-drained soil and full sunlight. Since the pungent leaves are very tasty, to maximize leaf production just pinch out flowering stalks as they appear. Leaving the flowers to bloom means you can harvest seeds at the end of the summer by tying paper bags over flower heads and hanging these upside down in a warm place.

Cilantro seeds were found in the tomb of the Egyptian pharaoh Tutankhamun, dating back to approximately 1300 BCE. To this day, in Egypt, the seeds and leaves are a popular ingredient in soups and bread making. In the Bible the taste of manna provided to the children of Israel by God is compared to cilantro seeds. The Romans are likely to have brought the herb to Britain and it is now grown in many countries.

SEE ALSO
Fennel, ginger, black pepper, turmeric, cinnamon

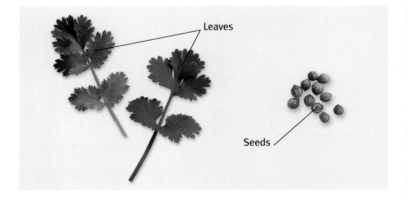

Leaves

Seeds

CILANTRO

Coriandrum sativum

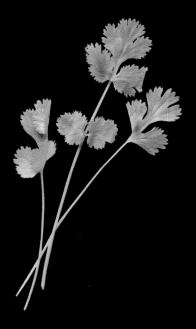

PARTS OF PLANT USED
Leaves and seeds

ACTIVE INGREDIENTS
Leaves: tannins, sugar and vitamin C; seeds: volatile oil

COMMERCIALLY AVAILABLE AS
Fresh leaves, dried seeds, cough medicine, essential oil (from seeds)

ACTIONS
Antispasmodic, digestive tonic

USED TO TREAT
Gas, indigestion: infusion of fresh leaves taken 2–3 times daily eases painful gas and helps to digest fatty foods.
Stress-related digestive upsets: 3 drops of essential oil added to 2 teaspoons of sunflower oil massaged clockwise into the abdomen helps to calm anxiety-related indigestion.
Muscular aches and pains: 4 drops of essential oil added to 2 teaspoons of sunflower oil and massaged into affected areas twice daily eases pain and improves circulation.

CULINARY USE
Chopped fresh leaves make a delicious garnish for curry dishes and can be added to green salads or mixed into dressings. The seeds are used in curries, chutneys, pickles, and in some bread and cake recipes.

SAFETY INFORMATION
No issues

CRATEGUS OXYACANTHA
• HAWTHORN

A deciduous, thorny shrub with dense branches, hawthorn can grow up to 30 ft (10 m) tall and can live to a very great age. Its soft green leaves are wedge-shaped and deeply lobed, with tufts of silken hairs where they join the main stem. Hawthorn is widely distributed throughout northern Europe, thriving in scrubland, woods, ditches, or along riverbanks. Its strong-scented flowers traditionally bloom in May—hence its common name "mayblossom"—and are white, leading to another common name, "whitethorn." The berries ("haws") are barrel-shaped and bright red in color. They usually ripen for picking in early fall; another common name for the shrub used to be "bread and cheese tree" because the berries were picked and eaten for energy by people who had to walk for long distances.

Hundreds of years ago in Britain, the first of May would be widely celebrated as a festival, with different kinds of rituals to welcome the fruitful growing season of late spring and summer. In villages, the prettiest girl was crowned "Queen of the May" and carried a wand made of flowering hawthorn, as well as wearing a crown made of mayblossom or hawthorn blooms. In these days of climate change it is not unusual to see hawthorn in blossom in late January or early February, much earlier than in ancient times.

SEE ALSO

Lavender, melissa, St. John's wort, German camomile, yarrow

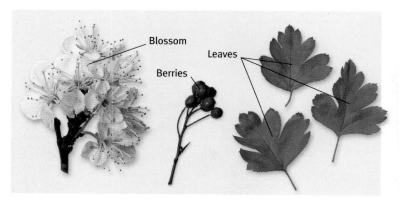

Blossom

Berries

Leaves

HAWTHORN

Crategus oxyacantha

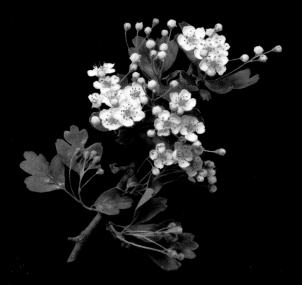

PARTS OF PLANT USED
Flowers, leaves, berries

ACTIVE INGREDIENTS
Glycosides, saponins, tannins

COMMERCIALLY AVAILABLE AS
Tablets, tincture

ACTIONS
Cardiac tonic, circulatory tonic, blood pressure regulator

USED TO TREAT
High blood pressure: tablets or tincture taken as directed help to regulate heart rate and reduce high blood pressure.
Poor circulation: tablets or tincture taken as directed improve coronary and peripheral blood flow.
Arrhythmia: tablets or tincture taken as directed have a regulatory effect on heart rate.

CULINARY USE
None

SAFETY INFORMATION
Do not take if you are under medical treatment or on drug medication for heart-related problems. It is advisable only to use hawthorn as a medicinal remedy under the guidance of a medical herbalist.

CURCUMA LONGA
● TURMERIC

A close botanical relative of ginger, turmeric is a perennial aromatic plant growing up to 4 ft (1.2 m) tall, with shiny, pointed pairs of lance-shaped leaves and spikes of yellow flowers. It has a yellow-colored, fleshy, tuberous root that is boiled, dried, and powdered before being used as a spice or medicinal ingredient, particularly in India. An attractive plant, it can be grown in pots in conservatories or greenhouses in cooler climates; it needs moist and well-nourished soil, a humid atmosphere, and a minimum temperature of 45°F (7°C). Once plants take, they can be propagated by dividing clumped roots and replanting them.

In India, turmeric is a classic cooking spice and traditional medicinal remedy. In Ayurveda, it is used as an anti-inflammatory remedy, and also to purify the blood and rid the intestines of parasites. Recent Indian scientific research has confirmed its beneficial effects on the intestines, even suggesting that turmeric's popularity in the diet may explain the low incidence of bowel cancer in India. The root is also used as a yellow dye as an alternative to saffron, which is very expensive.

SEE ALSO
Cinnamon, cardamom, ginger, garlic, black pepper

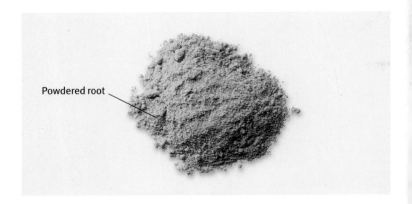

Powdered root

TURMERIC
Curcuma longa

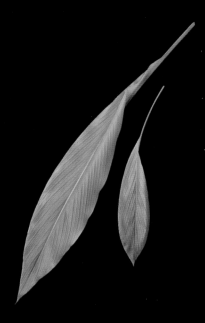

PART OF PLANT USED
Roots

ACTIVE INGREDIENTS
Iron, potassium, starch, vitamin C,
volatile oil

COMMERCIALLY AVAILABLE AS
Dried root (spice), essential oil,
ointment, tablets

ACTIONS
Antibiotic, diuretic, anti-inflammatory,
possibly antitumoral

USED TO TREAT
Diarrhea, sluggish digestion: tablets
taken as directed ease spasms.
Coughs, colds, sore throats: ointment,
or 3 drops of essential oil added to 2
teaspoons of sunflower oil massaged
into the chest warms the area and
supports the immune system.
Anemia: in traditional Indian medicine,
half a teaspoon of turmeric powder
infused in 7 fl oz (200 ml) of warm milk
can be drunk twice daily as an iron tonic.
Wounds, cuts, problem skin: 4 drops of
essential oil added to 2 teaspoons of
sunflower oil applied twice daily speeds
healing and discourages infection.

CULINARY USE
In Indian curry paste and powder mixes
for meat and vegetable dishes; also to
color rice.

SAFETY INFORMATION
No issues; if diarrhea persists seek
medical advice.

CYMBOPOGON CITRATUS
• LEMONGRASS

This aromatic grass grows in tall clumps up to 5 ft (1.5 m) high. It produces long, straight, strongly lemon-scented leaves, due to an aromatic ingredient in its volatile oil called "citral." It is native to countries such as Thailand, India, and Malaysia, where it thrives in a hot, moist environment. In cooler climates it can be grown as an exotic plant in pots in greenhouses or conservatories, provided the temperature does not fall below 45°F (7°C). It requires moist, very well-drained soil, regular doses of a good fertilizer, and high humidity—leaves need regular spraying to stop them drying out.

Lemongrass is widely cultivated throughout the Far East, where it is used medicinally to help lower fevers, including malaria, as well as to treat digestive or stress-related conditions. It has grown in popularity in the west over the past 20 years thanks to the spread of Thai and Indian cuisine, in which lemongrass adds a fresh flavor. In aromatherapy, the essential oil is used in massage to help muscular aches and pains and soothe depression; it is also a very popular natural fragrance in soaps, bath products, and perfumery.

SEE ALSO
Melissa, spearmint, peppermint, lemon verbena, bitter orange

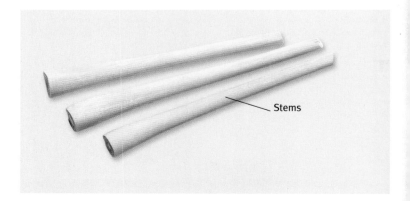

Stems

LEMONGRASS

Cymbopogon citratus

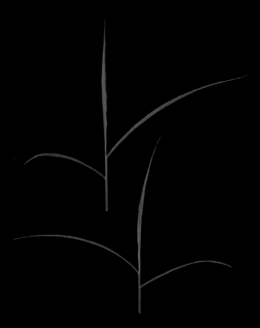

PART OF PLANT USED
Leaves

ACTIVE INGREDIENTS
Volatile oil

COMMERCIALLY AVAILABLE AS
Essential oil, fresh leaves

ACTIONS
Digestive tonic, antispasmodic, rubefacient

USED TO TREAT
Muscular aches and pains, poor circulation: 2 drops of essential oil in 2 teaspoons of sunflower oil massaged into affected areas eases pain and stimulates the circulation.
Indigestion, especially due to emotional stress: 2 drops of essential oil in 2 teaspoons of sunflower oil massaged clockwise into the abdomen twice daily calms anxiety and improves regularity.
Mental tiredness and depression: the aroma of two drops of essential oil on a Kleenex, inhaled, or two drops added to a vaporizer, uplifts low moods and encourages a positive attitude.

CULINARY USE
Fresh lower stems, chopped, are used as an important flavoring in Malaysian, Thai, and Indian cookery.

SAFETY INFORMATION
The essential oil should not be used on people with allergy-prone or sensitive skin, on damaged skin, or on children under the age of 10.

DAUCUS CAROTA
• CARROT

Originally this plant was the wild carrot with a small, white, pungent root, quite different to the large orange root of the sweeter-tasting carrot used in cooking today. The orange subspecies has been bred using horticultural crossing over hundreds of years. Carrot is a biennial herb up to 3 ft (1 m) tall, with wispy leaves, dense umbels of whitish-pink flowers that become flat seeds, and thick tap roots. It thrives in sandy, well-drained soil and needs full sun. The leaves and top part of the plant can be picked in late spring for infusions, and the seeds can be collected and dried at the end of summer.

The wild carrot, with its hot-tasting white root, was mentioned by the Roman scientist Pliny in the 1st century CE, and it is mentioned in writings on cookery from the 2nd century CE. Carrots have been cultivated throughout Europe since ancient Greek times and were introduced to Britain during the reign of Queen Elizabeth I. The now more familiar orange root vegetable contains several nutrients, including vitamin C, beta-carotene, sugars and minerals. Wild carrots are more medicinally potent than modern cultivated varieties, however, the leaves and seeds of cultivated species are more widely used today.

SEE ALSO
Angelica, fennel, peppermint, juniper, grapefruit

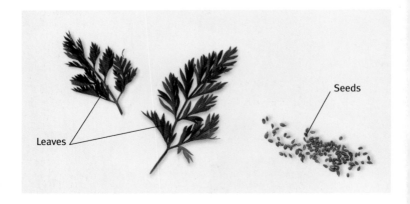

Leaves

Seeds

CARROT
Daucus carota

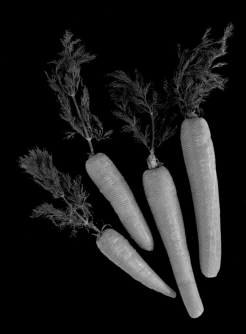

PARTS OF PLANT USED
Leaves, seeds

ACTIVE INGREDIENTS
Alkaloids (leaves), volatile oil (seeds)

COMMERCIALLY AVAILABLE AS
Essential oil (from seeds), tea, juice

ACTIONS
Antispasmodic, digestive tonic, diuretic

USED TO TREAT
Fluid retention, urinary tract infections: an infusion of fresh leaves taken twice a day acts as a mild diuretic, helping the body to excrete excess fluid.
Indigestion, gas, bloating: 2 drops of carrot-seed essential oil in 1 teaspoon of sunflower oil massaged clockwise into the abdomen twice daily eases painful gas and indigestion spasms.
Insomnia: 2 drops of carrot seed essential oil in a warm bathtub has a soothing, relaxing effect on the mind.

CULINARY USE
Carrots are popular eaten either raw or cooked. Fresh carrot juice is packed with pro-vitamin A, vitamin C, and minerals; drinking 6 fl oz (200 ml) of fresh carrot and apple juice combined in equal measure daily is an effective digestive and liver tonic.

SAFETY INFORMATION
No issues

DIOSCOREA VILLOSA
• WILD YAM

This perennial climbing plant has heart-shaped, vibrant green leaves, and produces only male or female flowers on a single plant, so both sexes have to be grown together if seed is required. Wild yam thrives in full sun and moist soil. It can grow up to 6ft (3 m) tall and flowers in September and October. It is native to eastern North America, from New England to Minnesota and Ontario, and south to Virginia and Texas; a related species grows in Mexico. It has a thick fleshy root called a "tuber," and this is the active medicinal part. Roots are dug up and dried for medicinal use and should not be stored for more than a year, as they lose their potency over time.

Wild yam and other members of the same plant family contain a substance called "diosgenin" in the roots, and this is a natural plant-steroid precursor of the hormone progesterone. This has led to the development of some very important drugs, such as the contraceptive pill, as well as medication for asthma and arthritis.

SEE ALSO
Agnus castus, sage, black cohosh, clary sage, Lady's mantle

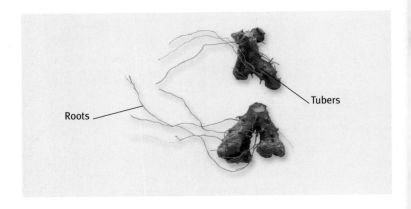

Tubers

Roots

WILD YAM

Dioscorea villosa

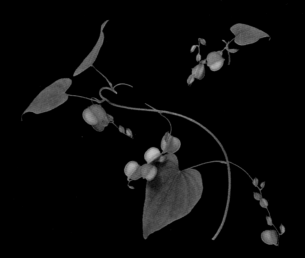

PART OF PLANT USED
Dried root

ACTIVE INGREDIENTS
Alkaloids, phytosterols, steroidal saponins, starch, tannins

COMMERCIALLY AVAILABLE AS
Capsules, tincture, cream

ACTIONS
Anti-inflammatory, antispasmodic, hormone regulating, nervous restorative

USED TO TREAT
Menstrual cramps, PMS, menopausal symptoms: tablets or tincture taken as directed calm period pain; cream applied daily under the arms, over the breasts, and abdomen eases hot flashes.

Gas, colic, abdominal cramps: tablets or tincture taken as directed ease cramping in the bowel, releasing trapped gas.
Nervousness, emotional stress: tablets or tincture taken as directed calm the nervous system and improve relaxation.
Rheumatoid arthritis (inflammatory stage): capsules or tincture taken as directed can be anti-inflammatory.

CULINARY USE
None

SAFETY INFORMATION
Only commercial preparations from the root are recommended. Not recommended for women with a history of estrogen-dependent cancer, or men with prostate cancer. Avoid in pregnancy and when breast-feeding.

ECHINACEA PURPUREA
• ECHINACEA

A perennial herb up to 4 ft (1.2 m) tall, echinacea grows from a thick root called a rhizome. It produces vigorous, bright green, lance-shaped leaves, and its flowers are deep pink with a daisy-like shape and a raised conical center—giving it the common name "purple cone flower." It grows wild in prairie or grassland regions and requires rich, well-drained soil in sun or partial shade. Cutting back the flowers as they fade encourages new blooms throughout the summer. It can be grown from seed in the spring, or propagated by digging up existing plants and dividing the root clumps in half and replanting them.

Echinacea is native to the United States where it was used extensively by many Native American tribes as a medicinal plant to heal wounds, treat snakebites, ease the pain of toothache, and as a general antiseptic. Early settlers adopted echinacea too, using the plant to help immunize against infections. Modern scientific research has confirmed echinacea's immune-boosting properties, and it is used in medical herbal practice as an antiviral to help immune-related problems, and as a blood-purifying skin treatment for recurring skin infections such as acne and boils.

SEE ALSO
Garlic, cardamom, black pepper, tea tree, lemon

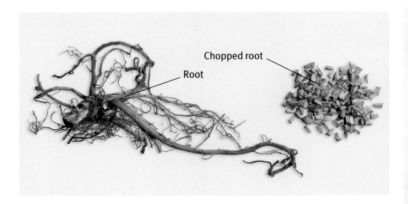

Chopped root

Root

ECHINACEA
Echinacea purpurea

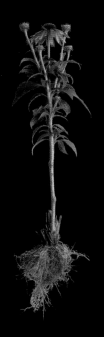

PART OF PLANT USED
Roots

ACTIVE INGREDIENTS
Fatty acids, inulin, plant sterols, polysaccharides, resin, volatile oil

COMMERCIALLY AVAILABLE AS
Tablets, capsules, tincture, tea (from flowers), ointment

ACTIONS
Antiseptic, antiviral, immune boosting

USED TO TREAT
Cold, influenza, viral infections: capsules, tablets, or tincture taken as directed stimulate the immune system.
Boils, pimples, acne: ointment applied twice daily heals infected areas; tablets, capsules, or tincture can be taken as directed as a blood-cleansing treatment.
Cuts, wounds, skin infections: ointment applied twice daily encourages wound healing and fights infection.
Inflamed or sore gums: tincture measured into water as directed, used as a mouthwash twice daily, soothes pain, reduces inflammation, and heals minor infections.

CULINARY USE
None

SAFETY INFORMATION
Echinacea should not be taken for more than three months at a time because its efficacy diminishes with prolonged use; if in doubt, always consult a qualified medical herbalist.

ELETTARIA CARDAMOMUM
• CARDAMOM

Cardamom is botanically related to ginger, and both plants look very similar. It has a large, fleshy root called a "rhizome," which produces elegant, lance-shaped leaves on stalks growing 6–8 ft (2–3 m) tall. Its flowers are small, with yellow and violet petals, produced at the base of the plant. These become small green pods containing shiny, black, aromatic seeds. Cardamom is native to countries such as India, but it will grow in cooler climates in a greenhouse or conservatory, with a minimum temperature of 64°F (18°C), in well-drained, rich soil and partial shade. It can be grown from seed or by dividing clumps of roots and replanting.

Cardamom has been traded as an important spice throughout India and the Far East for centuries. In India, where the plant originates, it is called *"elattari,"* which accounts for the first part of its botanical name. Cardamom has been used in Indian Ayurvedic medicine for centuries as a circulatory, respiratory, and adrenal tonic. The ancient Greeks and Romans included it in early lists of exotic spice ingredients.

SEE ALSO
Cilantro, ginger, turmeric, garlic, cayenne pepper

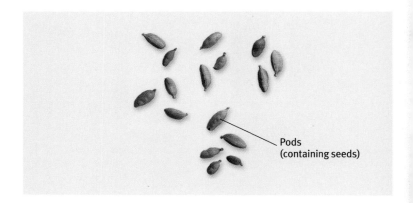

Pods
(containing seeds)

CARDAMOM

Elettaria cardamomum

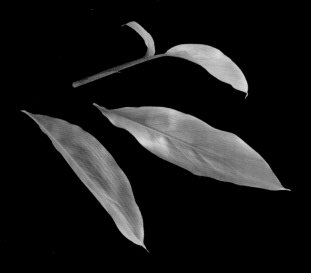

PART OF PLANT USED
Seeds

ACTIVE INGREDIENTS
Mucilage, resin, volatile oil

COMMERCIALLY AVAILABLE AS
Essential oil, pods (spice), tablets, capsules

ACTIONS
Antispasmodic, circulation stimulating, digestive tonic, immune tonic

USED TO TREAT
Colds, influenza: 2 drops of essential oil in 1 teaspoon of sunflower oil massaged twice daily into the upper chest helps boost immunity and fight viral infections.
Coughs: 2 drops of essential oil in 1 teaspoon of sunflower oil massaged into the upper chest twice daily eases coughing.
Poor circulation, rheumatism: 4 drops of essential oil in 2 teaspoons of sunflower oil massaged into affected areas twice daily improves circulation.
Indigestion: commercial tablets taken as directed, or an infusion made with 1 teaspoon of seeds, drunk twice daily, to ease pain and improve digestive function.

CULINARY USE
Used in curry powder with cumin, black pepper, chili, ginger, and cilantro. In India it is drunk as a spicy tea, and used to flavor sweets and ice creams.

SAFETY INFORMATION
No issues

EQUISETUM ARVENSE
• HORSETAIL FERN

This is a vigorous, fast-spreading, perennial plant up to 20 in (50 cm) in height. It has tough stems, which produce cones at the tips, releasing spores. This method of reproduction is the same as that employed by ferns. Its mass of green stems is sterile. Horsetail fern grows best in moist conditions in sun or partial shade. It can be propagated by division of roots, but be warned—if you plant it in your garden, it is impossible to eradicate once it has spread. If you want to use the plant yourself, it is best to find a regular wild source away from traffic, such as on waste ground, harvesting in June or July and drying for later use.

Horsetail ferns are a separate plant family, closely related botanically to ferns. Millions of years ago, during the period known as the Carboniferous era, the ancestors of modern horsetail plants grew as tall as trees. Today, horsetail ferns are found growing wild on waste ground, in woods and wet meadows all over Europe. Sadly, this plant is often regarded as a weed, yet it is a very efficient and useful healing remedy.

SEE ALSO
Yarrow, myrrh, red clover, German camomile, saw palmetto

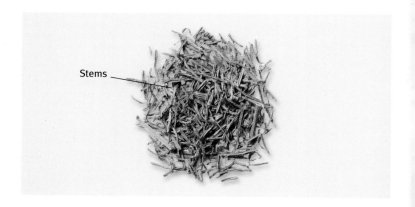

Stems

HORSETAIL FERN

Equisetum arvense

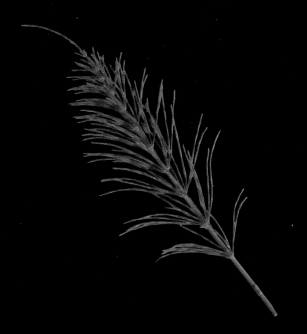

PART OF PLANT USED
Green stems

ACTIVE INGREDIENTS
Alkaloids, flavonoids, minerals, saponins, silica

COMMERCIALLY AVAILABLE AS
Capsules, tablets, tincture

ACTIONS
Astringent, diuretic, skin and hair nutrient

USED TO TREAT
Bleeding (fast flowing from wounds): a strong infusion of fresh leaves and stems slows bleeding in the first stages of recovery from injury.
Prostate/bladder disorders: capsules, tablets, or tincture taken as directed act as a tonic to the bladder, prostate gland and urinary system.
Rough skin, wounds, brittle nails, thinning hair: tablets, capsules, or tincture taken as directed bring silica into the system, which is vital as a building block for new skin cells.
Anemia, general lack of energy: mineral-rich horsetail fern, taken as capsules, tablets, or tincture as directed, is an excellent all-round tonic for the system.

CULINARY USE
None

SAFETY INFORMATION
Though horsetail fern can be used as a first-aid herb for bleeding, if symptoms persist, seek medical advice.

ERICA VULGARIS
• HEATHER

A tough shrub with stems that grow up to 2 ft (60 cm) high, heather has tiny, needle-like, overlapping leaves, creating a dense mat of foliage. It produces spikes of tiny, deep-pink flowers, typically from July to September, followed by small, round berries. Although many ornamental horticultural varieties exist, only the wild species is medicinally potent. It grows extensively on bogs, moors, hillsides and heathland, for example in Scotland or on the Yorkshire Moors in England. It is native to northern Europe, North Africa and eastern North America. It can be cultivated from seed and requires full sun and acidic soil with plenty of water—it particularly thrives in a rock garden. Heather has the added benefit of attracting butterflies, bees, ladybugs, and other beneficial insects to a garden. Flowers can be picked in late summer and used fresh or hung upside down in bunches to dry before storing for later use.

Wild heather has a varied history of use in northern Europe—for example, it was used to make strong ale, honey, an orange-yellow dye for cloth, and medicine. In western herbal tradition heather is valued as a detoxifying remedy for the kidneys and urinary tract, as well as for its soothing effects on rheumatism.

SEE ALSO
Devil's claw, cardamom, cayenne pepper, juniper, eucalyptus

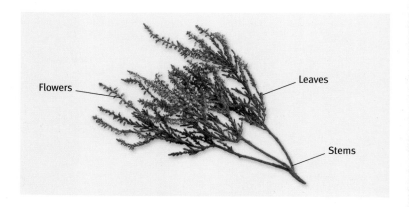

Flowers

Leaves

Stems

HEATHER
Erica vulgaris

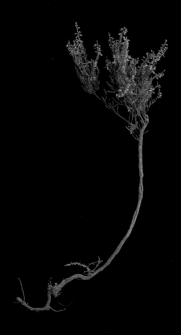

PART OF PLANT USED
Fresh flowering tops

ACTIVE INGREDIENTS
Arbutin, citric acid, glycosides, resin, tannins

COMMERCIALLY AVAILABLE AS
Tea, tincture

ACTIONS
Anti-inflammatory, detoxifying, diuretic, sedative

USED TO TREAT
Rheumatism, osteoarthritis, backache: fresh flowering tops made into macerated oil or ointment (see pages 298–9) applied twice daily to affected parts eases pain and stiffness; a handful of fresh flowering tops tied in a muslin bag can be added to a hot bathtub for pain relief.
Muscular aches and pains, physical tiredness: a handful of fresh flowering tops tied in a muslin bag added to a hot bathtub relaxes aching muscles and soothes the mind.
Fluid retention, urinary tract infections, prostatitis: tea can be drunk twice daily or tincture taken as directed to ease irritation and discomfort, and release the flow of urine.

CULINARY USE
None

SAFETY INFORMATION
No issues

ERYTHREA CENTAURIUM
• CENTAURY

This annual herb grows up to 12 in (30 cm) tall, with a tough, erect stem, and pairs of oval leaves joined directly at the base. It produces small clusters of deep pink flowers, followed by small berries. It is native throughout Europe, thriving on waste ground, especially in dry, grassy locations. It is cultivated for medicinal use in central and eastern Europe. This herb is closely related to yellow gentian (*Gentiana lutea*, see pages 124–5); both are bitter tonics used for liver and gall-bladder support. The flowering tops need to be harvested in high summer, usually July, just before the flowers are in full bloom; the herb is then dried to preserve the active ingredients.

Many ancient European herbals mention centaury—it has been in use for hundreds of years as an appetite stimulant and digestive tonic, as well as a cure for fever (one of its old-fashioned names was "feverwort.") Anglo-Saxon herbalists regarded it as one of the best cures for poison in the body. Another ancient medical name for this herb was "*Fel terrae*" which translates as "gall of the Earth," because of its extremely bitter taste. Throughout Europe, centaury and yellow gentian are still used in the making of bitter liqueurs, which, if taken in small doses after heavy meals, help to prevent indigestion.

SEE ALSO
Yellow gentian, fennel, grapefruit, turmeric, angelica

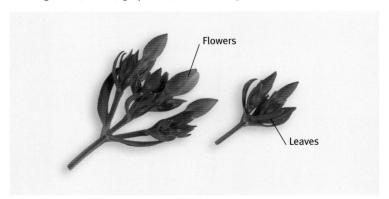

Flowers

Leaves

CENTAURY

Erythrea centaurium

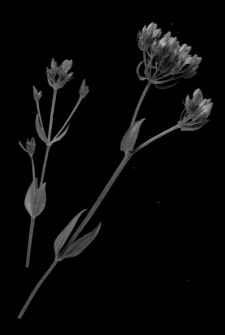

PART OF PLANT USED
Flowering tops

ACTIVE INGREDIENTS
Alkaloids, bitter glycosides, phenolic acids, tannins

COMMERCIALLY AVAILABLE AS
Tablets, tincture

ACTIONS
Anti-inflammatory, digestive tonic, laxative, liver and gall-bladder tonic

USED TO TREAT
Poor liver function, liver and gall-bladder problems: tablets or tincture taken as directed increase secretions from the liver and gallbladder to aid digestion.

Indigestion, especially of rich or fatty foods: tablets or tincture taken as directed gently release the bowel and increase digestive secretions.
Fevers: tablets or tincture taken as directed reduce body temperature.
Rheumatism and gout: tablets or tincture taken as directed have a cleansing and detoxifying effect on the body.

CULINARY USE
None

SAFETY INFORMATION
Persistent or severe digestive upsets should be referred to a doctor or qualified medical herbalist.

EUCALYPTUS GLOBULUS
• EUCALYPTUS

There are around 300 species of eucalyptus, and this one is a very tall tree, able to reach heights of up to 300 ft (100 m) at full spread. It has pale bark, which tends to peel away, and the wood is aromatic. The leaves are very pungent, usually slightly darker on the upper surface and pale beneath; they contain sacs filled with volatile oil. The flowers are whitish, followed by round berries. Eucalyptus trees prefer hot climates but can be planted in temperate gardens provided the temperature does not fall below 23°F (−5°C). They require well-drained soil and full sun and will out-compete other plants and trees for water, because they are experts at survival in their harsh native environment—the outback of Australia. In North Africa and southern Europe they have been deliberately planted in marshy areas to reclaim land and reduce the mosquito population.

Eucalyptus essential oil has been produced on a large commercial scale since the 19th century; it is commonly used in the pharmaceutical industry to make cold and cough remedies and ointments for muscular aches.

SEE ALSO
Peppermint, rosemary, tea tree, manuka, lemon

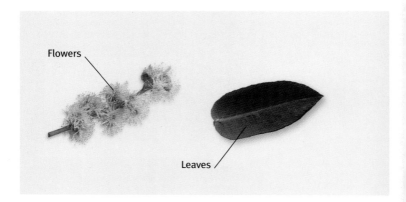

Flowers

Leaves

EUCALYPTUS
Eucalyptus globulus

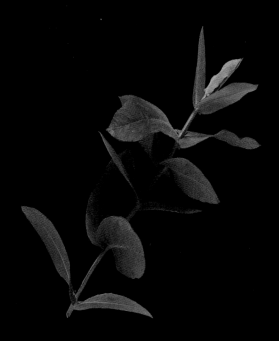

PART OF PLANT USED
Leaves

ACTIVE INGREDIENTS
Volatile oil

COMMERCIALLY AVAILABLE AS
Essential oil, cough medicine, lozenges, massage balm, ointment

ACTIONS
Antiseptic, expectorant, vulnerary

USED TO TREAT
Cuts, grazes, wounds: infusion of fresh leaves can be used to cleanse and disinfect affected areas; ointment can be applied as directed to speed healing.
Sinusitis, colds: add 2 drops of essential oil to a bowl of boiling water and inhale the vapor for 10 minutes to improve breathing; lozenges taken as directed also ease airways.
Coughs: 2 drops of essential oil added to 1 teaspoon of sunflower oil massaged twice daily into the chest eases coughs; cough medicine can be taken as directed.
Muscular aches and pains: 4 drops of essential oil added to 2 teaspoons of sunflower oil massaged into affected areas twice daily eases pain and stiffness and improves movement; massage balm can be used as directed.

CULINARY USE
None

SAFETY INFORMATION
Infusion of fresh leaves or the essential oil should not be used on sensitive skin.

EUGENIA CARYOPHYLLATA
• CLOVE

Clove trees grow to 65 ft (20 m) in height. They have a gray bark, dark green, shiny leaves, and aromatic green buds which, if they are not picked, will turn into dark red flowers. The dried unripe buds are the "cloves" sold commercially. Trees need to be at least six years old before the cloves can be harvested to ensure maximum potency. Clove trees are originally native to Indonesia and require full tropical conditions—fertile soil, high humidity, and hot temperatures. They will not grow in cooler climates.

Early Persian and Arab traders who established trade routes to the Indonesian islands probably introduced cloves to Europe. The Latin name "*caryophyllata*" dates back to the Roman writer Pliny in the 1st century CE, who knew them as "*caryophyllon*." In the 16th century they were carried around as a popular protection against the plague, stuffed with other spices into the leather face masks worn by physicians. The name "clove" comes from the French "*clou*," meaning "nail," because of the shape of the spice.

SEE ALSO
Cardamom, ginger, garlic, cayenne pepper, black pepper

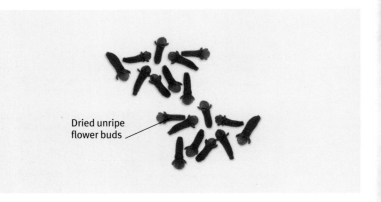

Dried unripe
flower buds

CLOVE

Eugenia caryophyllata

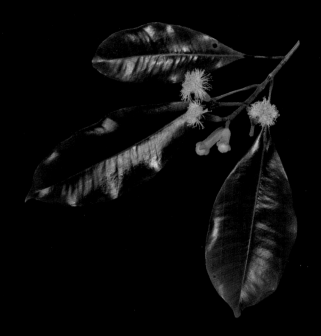

PART OF PLANT USED
Dried unripe flower buds (clove nails)

ACTIVE INGREDIENTS
Volatile oil

COMMERCIALLY AVAILABLE AS
Cough medicine, essential oil, whole or ground spice

ACTIONS
Antiseptic, antiviral, circulation stimulant, expectorant

USED TO TREAT
Indigestion, nausea, gas: infuse 4 cloves in 7 fl oz (200 ml) boiling water and drink twice daily to ease gas.
Toothache: soften 1 clove by soaking it in 4 tablespoons of boiling water for 10 minutes, then place it between the teeth to numb pain.
Colds, influenza, coughs: add 2 drops of essential oil to a small bowl of boiling water and inhale the vapor for 20 minutes to help unblock airways and ease the chest; commercial medicine can be taken as directed to ease coughs.

CULINARY USE
Cloves complement cooked ham or pork dishes and are essential in mulled wine. they are delicious cooked with apples or added to pickles and chutneys. They are also used as a spice in Indian cuisine.

SAFETY INFORMATION
Essential oil should not be applied to individuals with sensitive skin, or to children under the age of five.

EUPHRASIA OFFICINALIS
• EYEBRIGHT

This annual herb has thin, wiry stems up to 12 in (30 cm) in height and small, toothed, round leaves. It grows in a parasitic way, attaching itself with suckers to the roots of other plants, particularly grasses, to obtain nutrients (although it does no harm to the host plant and dies back in the fall). It therefore needs to be sown near or in grass. Eyebright's delicate flowers are white with vein-like streaks of purple around a yellow center— these are the medicinally active part of the plant. The flowering tops are best harvested in July or August when the plant is in full flower; they can be used fresh or carefully dried and stored for up to one year.

The botanical name of the plant, "*Euphrasia*," is of Greek origin, derived from the name of one of the Three Graces, Euphrosyne, who brought joy and laughter—perhaps because the plant has been celebrated for centuries for its soothing and calming properties, especially when applied to eye problems. In the 16th century, eyebright tea, eyebright wine, and eyebright ale were commonly drunk as health-giving tonics. The 17th-century English herbalist Nicholas Culpeper used this herb to help poor eyesight, and improve brain and memory function.

SEE ALSO

Cornflower, Roman camomile, yarrow, white horehound, myrtle

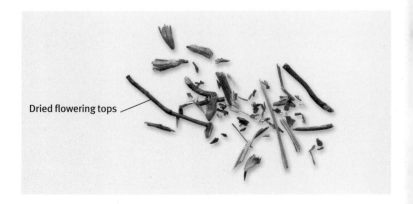

Dried flowering tops

112

EYEBRIGHT

Euphrasia officinalis

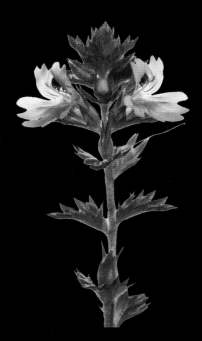

PART OF PLANT USED
Flowering tops

ACTIVE INGREDIENTS
Glycosides, saponins, resin, tannins, volatile oil

COMMERCIALLY AVAILABLE AS
Capsules, tablets, tincture

ACTIONS
Anti-inflammatory, skin soothing, cooling

USED TO TREAT
Hay fever, allergic rhinitis: infusion of fresh flowering tops taken 2–3 times daily soothes respiratory passages; capsules, tablets, or tincture taken as directed can have a preventive effect.

Catarrh, coughs, chest congestion: capsules or tablets taken as directed help to clear congestion in the chest and improve breathing.
Eye soreness, inflammation, itching: an infusion of fresh flowering tops, cooled, can be used as an eyewash to soothe the eyes, or soaked cotton balls can be applied to cool and calm the area.
Sore throats, sore gums: an infusion of fresh flowering tops, cooled, can be used twice daily as an anti-inflammatory mouthwash and gargle.

CULINARY USE
None

SAFETY INFORMATION
No issues

FILIPENDULA ULMARIA
• MEADOWSWEET

This plant has a tough, erect stem and grows up to 4 ft (1.2 m) tall. Its leaves are serrated, typically dark green on the upper surface and pale below, with an almond-like aroma. Meadowsweet produces flat clusters of tiny, creamy white flowers with a strong, sweet smell. It thrives in damp woods and meadows, boggy places, and on riverbanks. It is found growing wild all over Europe, and should be collected in high summer, usually July, when it is in flower. It can be used fresh or dried and stored for up to a year.

Because of meadowsweet's pleasant smells—different in the flowers and leaves—it was popular in medieval times as a "strewing herb," thrown on the ground for people to walk on to release the aroma. It was also used to flavor mead, an alcoholic drink made from fermented honey. In the 1890s in Germany, aspirin was originally synthesized from willow bark and meadowsweet—both are natural sources of salicylic acid, the main analgesic ingredient, which becomes acetylsalicylic acid in the synthetic form. Some herbalists maintain that because meadowsweet contains buffering ingredients such as tannins, these can help prevent the internal bleeding that can be associated with synthetic aspirin—the whole herb with all its ingredients in balance is less invasive than a synthetic copy of one key ingredient.

SEE ALSO
White willow, German camomile, valerian, melissa, lavender

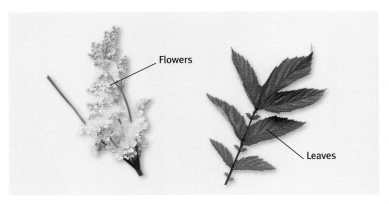

Flowers

Leaves

MEADOWSWEET

Filipendula ulmaria

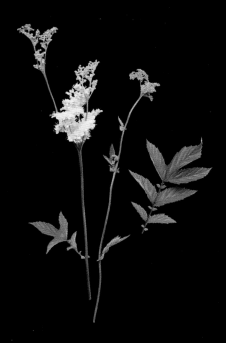

PARTS OF PLANT USED
Flowers and leaves

ACTIVE INGREDIENTS
Flavonoids, mucilage, salicylates, sugar, tannins, vitamin C, volatile oil

COMMERCIALLY AVAILABLE AS
Tablets, tincture

ACTIONS
Antiseptic, analgesic, antiacidic, anti-inflammatory, diuretic

USED TO TREAT
Headaches, neuralgia: tablets or tincture taken as directed soothe pain and ease inflammation.
Rheumatism, arthritis: tablets or tincture taken as directed calm inflammation and soothe pain associated with rheumatism and arthritis.
Indigestion, heartburn, diarrhea, gastritis: tablets or tincture taken as directed help to neutralize excess acid in the stomach.

CULINARY USE
None

SAFETY INFORMATION
Best avoided by people sensitive to aspirin, though the herb is unlikely to have internal side effects. If in doubt, check with a doctor or medical herbalist.

FOENICULUM VULGARE
• FENNEL

This dramatic-looking biennial herb can grow up to 6 ft (2 m) tall, with long stems and feathery, aromatic foliage. Umbels of yellow flowers bloom in high summer. The seeds are ridged and yellow-green. Fennel can easily be grown from seed and requires sandy soil and full sun. Cut out the flowering stalks to encourage more leaves for culinary use, or leave the flowers to bloom for seed production. In late summer, tie paper bags around flower heads, cut them off, then hang them upside down until the seeds drop off.

In the 1st century CE the Roman writer Pliny recommended fennel for a whole range of physical disorders, including weight loss, due to its diuretic action. In the 12th century fennel was a favored herbal remedy in the medical writings of the German abbess, physician, and mystic, Hildegard of Bingen. She used it for toning the heart, improving the skin, bad breath, general detoxification, eye strain, stomach complaints, coughs, and runny noses.

SEE ALSO
Angelica, celery seed, cilantro, peppermint, spearmint

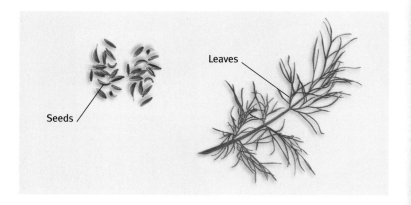

Leaves

Seeds

FENNEL

Foeniculum vulgare

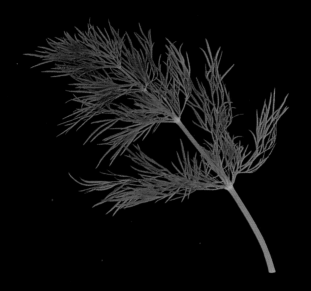

PART OF PLANT USED
Seeds

ACTIVE INGREDIENTS
Fatty acids, mucilage, proteins, sugar, volatile oil

COMMERCIALLY AVAILABLE AS
Capsules, tablets, tea, seeds, essential oil

ACTIONS
Antispasmodic, digestive tonic, diuretic, hormone regulator

USED TO TREAT
Indigestion, stomach ache, gas (especially after oily food): commercial tea or seed infusion can be drunk 2–3 times daily to ease spasm and nausea.
Fluid retention: 2 drops of essential oil added to 1 teaspoon of sunflower oil massaged into the affected area twice daily assists detoxification; tablets or capsules taken as directed are diuretic.
Sore gums, minor mouth infections: an infusion of seeds or commercial tea, cooled, can be used as a mouthwash to help soothe inflammation.

CULINARY USE
Fennel leaves add a strong aniseed flavor to oily fish dishes, and can be an aromatic garnish to soups, meat, and vegetable stews. The seeds can be chewed after a meal to help digestion.

SAFETY INFORMATION
In pregnancy, the seeds should not be swallowed or the essential oil used in massage.

FRAGARIA VESCA
• WILD STRAWBERRY

This perennial plant has a short fleshy rhizome, which produces long runners at soil level; these spread beyond the parent, take root, and become new plants. The leaves form in rosettes and have a trifoliate shape. White flowers arise directly from root level on long stalks and swell up to become the red fruit, which are very small and taste sharply sweet. The wild strawberry is the only species of strawberry with medicinal value. The common horticultural species, *Fragaria ananassa,* is a large-fruited hybrid of American origin, with many varieties, and its leaves have no active ingredients. Wild strawberries will grow easily in a garden, though they may be best contained in pots. They need well-drained soil in sun or partial shade, and lots of plant food. The leaves should be picked and dried in midsummer for medicinal use.

¹¹⁸ The name "strawberry" is probably derived from the Anglo-Saxon word "*streauberige*," which literally means "strewn berry" ("strewn" is an old English word meaning "tossed" or "thrown randomly"). This may refer to the haphazard appearance of the plant, as well as its long, trailing stems and method of spreading itself. The fruit is an excellent source of vitamin C.

SEE ALSO
Celery seed, fennel, red clover, lavender, aloe vera

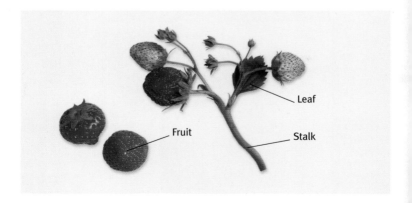

Leaf

Fruit

Stalk

WILD STRAWBERRY

Fragaria vesca

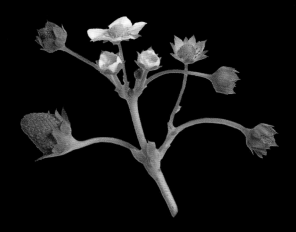

PARTS OF PLANT USED
Leaves, fruit

ACTIVE INGREDIENTS
Bitters, tannins, vitamin C, volatile oil

COMMERCIALLY AVAILABLE AS
Tea, tablets

ACTIONS
Astringent, diuretic

USED TO TREAT
Urinary-tract infections: tablets taken as directed, or an infusion of dried or fresh leaves has a diuretic effect, improving the flow of urine.
Indigestion: tablets taken as directed, or an infusion of fresh or dried leaves assists indigestion due to fatty foods.

Oily or combination skin: infusion of dried or fresh leaves, cooled, applied to the skin, tones open pores and clears excess oiliness.
Sunburn: a bowl of fresh wild or cultivated strawberries mashed to a pulp soothes and calms angry red skin.

CULINARY USE
Strawberry fruits (wild and cultivated) are an excellent source of vitamin C, particularly when eaten raw.

SAFETY INFORMATION
No issues

FUCUS VESICULOSIS
• KELP

Native to the coasts of northern Europe, this type of seaweed and some of its close relatives, such as _Fucus serratus_, are collected and made into the nutritional supplement known as kelp. _Fucus vesiculosis_ attaches itself to rocks with tough, woody roots developed from the base of the stalk. It produces brownish green fronds that can be up to 2 ft (60 cm) long. At the ends these divide into bifurcated branches with a tough, leathery texture and with small, swollen globules that contain the oval-shaped fruit. The entire plant is collected in June before it becomes too mature. For medicinal purposes, the seaweed has to be picked off the rocks while it is still rooted; if it is floating loose in the water, it will have lost many of its potent ingredients. It is then dried, traditionally in the sun, which makes it brittle and therefore easy to reduce to a powder, which is made into kelp tablets.

This type of seaweed was the original source of iodine, discovered in the early 1800s. Iodine is vital to the healthy function of the thyroid gland. Kelp is commonly taken as a supplement to support thyroid action and improve metabolism, while its high mineral content also means that it is a valuable nutritional tonic to the body.

SEE ALSO
Angelica, grapefruit, juniper, wild yam, silver birch

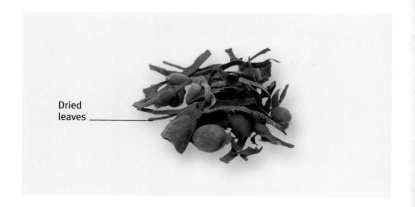

Dried
leaves _____

KELP
Fucus vesiculosis

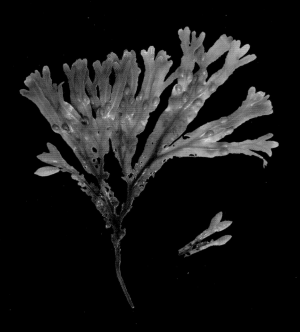

PART OF PLANT USED
Dried leaves

ACTIVE INGREDIENTS
Iodine, mucilage, potassium, volatile oil

COMMERCIALLY AVAILABLE AS
Tablets

ACTIONS
Anti-inflammatory, metabolic tonic

USED TO TREAT
Low thyroid function: tablets taken as directed help to tone and enhance the action of the thyroid gland.
Weight problems (if linked to low thyroid function): low thyroid function can lead to weight gain, so taking kelp tablets can correct metabolic imbalance.

Rheumatism, arthritis: commercial tablets taken as directed can have an anti-inflammatory effect, relieving pain and easing movement.

CULINARY USE
None for this kind of seaweed, though other species are used in cooking, for example nori in Japanese recipes.

SAFETY INFORMATION
If you are taking thyroxine or are under medical supervision for thyroid-related issues always consult your doctor before taking kelp.

GALIUM VERUM
• LADY'S BEDSTRAW

This perennial herb has wiry and erect, upright stems growing up to 3 ft (1 m) tall. Its vivid green leaves are narrow and arranged in groups of eight, radiating out from a common base. In July and August it produces bright yellow flowers with a honey-like scent. These turn into black berries at the end of the growing season. Lady's bedstraw thrives in sandy soils and on dry banks near the sea. It is common and widespread throughout Europe, including the British Isles. The flowering stems are the active medicinal part of the plant and need to be harvested in high summer, hung upside down, and dried before storage.

"Lady's bedstraw" is a common English name that describes one of this plant's past uses—as part of the stuffing of mattresses, probably because of its sweet smell. The leaves and stems of the plant also release a natural yellow dye, which in the past was used to color certain types of cheese bright yellow or orange. The leaves also curdle milk, so they were used in cheese-making, too—another old-fashioned name of this plant in English is "cheese rennet" (rennet is another substance that curdles milk). "*Galium*," part of the botanical name, is derived from the Greek word "*gala*," meaning milk. The roots of lady's bedstraw release a red dye, used at one time for coloring textiles.

SEE ALSO
Myrrh, yarrow, German camomile, calendula, bearberry/uva ursi

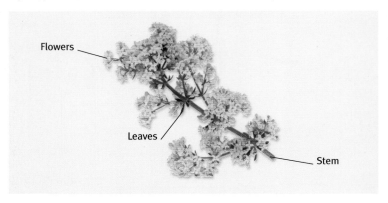

Flowers

Leaves

Stem

LADY'S BEDSTRAW

Galium verum

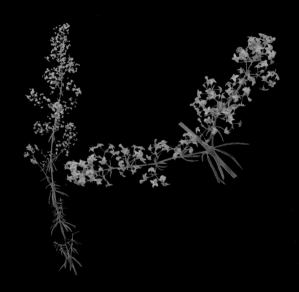

PART OF PLANT USED
Flowering tops

ACTIVE INGREDIENTS
Enzymes, glycosides, volatile oil

COMMERCIALLY AVAILABLE AS
Dried herb

ACTIONS
Antiseptic, antispasmodic, diuretic

USED TO TREAT
Wounds, ulcers, damaged skin: an infusion of the fresh or dried herb, cooled, applied to affected areas 2–3 times daily, has a disinfectant action and speeds wound healing.
Deep cuts, bleeding: an ointment made with the fresh or dried herb applied 2–3 times daily to the affected areas slows bleeding and helps wound healing.
Urinary tract infection and other minor urinary infections: an infusion of the fresh or dried herb drunk twice a day helps soothe irritation and improves the flow of urine.

CULINARY USE
None

SAFETY INFORMATION
No issues; however, regarding bleeding, if symptoms persist please seek medical help.

GENTIANA LUTEA
• YELLOW GENTIAN

This dramatic-looking herb grows from a thick, yellowish-brown root, sometimes up to 1 ft (30 cm) in length. The stem grows up to 3 ft (1 m) tall, with a pair of stiff, veined leaves arranged opposite each other at each node and joined at the base. Clusters of prominent yellow flowers form inside the leaves, making it seem as if the leaves are cups filled with blooms. Yellow gentian needs deep, rich soil, plenty of moisture, and strong sunlight for successful growth. Plants take up to three years to produce fully flowering stems, and the roots—the medicinally important part—are most potent once the plant has reached its flowering cycle. Yellow gentian is native to the Carpathian Mountains of eastern Europe, and is also found in France, Switzerland, Germany, and parts of central Europe. It is a protected species in the wild as it is becoming increasingly rare, but it can be grown in gardens as a spectacular ornamental plant.

124

The root of this plant has been used for centuries in countries such as France and Switzerland to produce "*liqueur de gentiane*," a digestive alcoholic drink, which, if taken in small amounts, acts as a very effective tonic to the digestive system and liver. The bitter compounds in yellow gentian are responsible for the beneficial gastric effects.

SEE ALSO

Centaury, peppermint, ginger, spearmint, turmeric

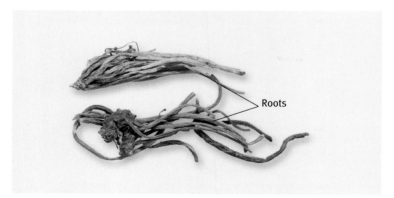

Roots

YELLOW GENTIAN

Gentiana lutea

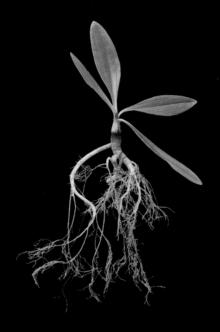

PART OF PLANT USED
Roots

ACTIVE INGREDIENTS
Alkaloids, bitter glycosides, sugar, volatile oil

COMMERCIALLY AVAILABLE AS
Tablets, tincture, liqueur

ACTIONS
Digestive tonic, liver and gallbladder tonic

USED TO TREAT
Poor appetite, sluggish digestion: 2 teaspoons (10 ml) of gentian liqueur taken before a meal stimulates gastric juices and sharpens appetite; tincture taken as directed has a similar effect.
Digestive nausea: 2 teaspoons (10 ml) of gentian liqueur relieves symptoms; tincture can also be taken as directed for the same effect.
Indigestion of fatty or oily foods: tablets or tincture taken as directed support the liver and gallbladder in the digestion of heavier meals.

CULINARY USE
None

SAFETY INFORMATION
Yellow gentian should not be taken by people suffering from duodenal or gastric ulcers.

GINKGO BILOBA
• GINKGO

This deciduous tree is actually a living fossil, belonging to a family that dates back more than 200 million years, to when dinosaurs roamed the Earth. Ginkgo trees can grow up to 100 ft (30 m) tall and 30 ft (10 m) wide, with sparse branches and an irregular growing habit. The bark of the tree is grooved, with a cork-like texture, and is highly resistant to disease, pests, fungi, and fire. Often, new stalks and leaves grow straight out of the trunk. The flat leaves are unusual, with a fan shape and several veins radiating from the stalk. Ginkgo trees are "dioecious," meaning that the male and female reproductive structures are produced on separate male and female trees. The fruits of the female tree, regarded as a delicacy in the Far East, have an extremely unpleasant smell—for this reason most ginkgos in parks tend to be male.

Ginkgo seeds have been used in traditional Chinese medicine for centuries to help asthma. In the past 20 years, scientific research, particularly in Germany, has revealed several important compounds in ginkgo leaves, suggesting it may improve memory function, have an antioxidant effect in the body, and an anti-allergic effect on asthma.

SEE ALSO

Rosemary, peppermint, myrtle, St. John's wort, lavender

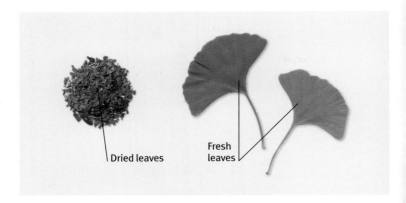

Dried leaves

Fresh leaves

GINKGO

Ginkgo biloba

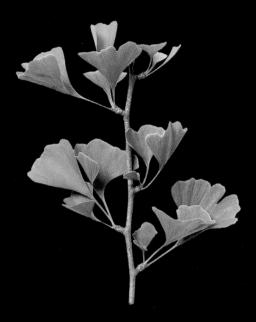

PART OF PLANT USED
Leaves

ACTIVE INGREDIENTS
Flavone glycosides, terpenes

COMMERCIALLY AVAILABLE AS
Capsules, tablets, tincture

ACTIONS
Antioxidant, antidepressant, cerebral circulation stimulant

USED TO TREAT
Age-related cognitive decline/ Alzheimer's disease: capsules, tablets, or tincture taken as directed for at least 12 weeks improve oxygen and blood flow to the brain, helping enhance memory and concentration.

Depression: tablets, capsules, or tincture taken as directed can help ease anxiety and mood-related symptoms.

Asthma: tablets, capsules, or tincture taken as directed may help to inhibit symptoms, particularly any allergic causes for asthma.

CULINARY USE
None

SAFETY INFORMATION
Indicated for conditions affecting older people who are likely to be on other types of medication—medical advice should always be sought for this group. Ginkgo should not be taken during pregnancy, breastfeeding, or in infancy. Avoid ginkgo if you are epileptic or taking any kind of anticoagulant medication.

GLYCYRRHIZA GLABRA
• LICORICE

This perennial shrub has a thick, woody, creeping rhizome, which is the active medicinal part of the plant. Above ground, it produces graceful, erect, branched stems up to 2 ft (60 cm) tall, with alternate long, oval leaves. The small flowers are blue-violet in color and arranged in tall spikes, becoming small pods that contain seeds. Licorice is found naturally all over Europe, in France, Italy, Germany, and as far afield as Russia and central Asia. It is now cultivated commercially worldwide. Licorice requires sandy soil and a great deal of moisture to thrive; it also needs strong summer temperatures to develop the roots. Plants must be a minimum of three years old before the roots are ready to be used medicinally, and the roots are generally harvested in the fall of the fourth growing season for maximum potency. They are then dried and ground into powder.

Licorice is one of the most widely researched medicinal herbs, with many useful properties. It contains a sweet ingredient called glycyrrhizin, which is about 50 times sweeter than sugar. Licorice is widely sold in herbal tablet combinations for digestive troubles, as well as in licorice confectionery.

SEE ALSO

Myrrh, turmeric, clove, Roman camomile, aloe vera

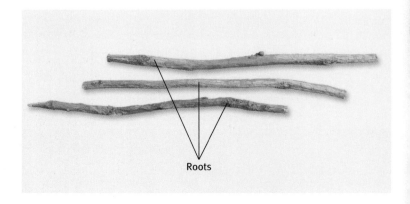

Roots

LICORICE

Glycyrrhiza glabra

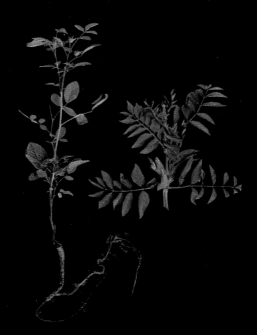

PART OF PLANT USED
Roots

ACTIVE INGREDIENTS
Glycosides, glycyrrhizin, saponins, starch, sugar, tannins, volatile oil

COMMERCIALLY AVAILABLE AS
Tablets, capsules, tea, dried root, confectionery.

ACTIONS
Anti-inflammatory, antispasmodic, demulcent, expectorant, laxative

USED TO TREAT
Coughs: tablets, capsules, or tincture taken as directed calm coughing.
Indigestion, poor assimilation, constipation: tablets, capsules, or tincture taken as directed, or tea drunk 2–3 times daily ease irregular spasms in the gut and help restore bowel rhythm.
Gastric ulceration: licorice is demulcent, meaning it has a soothing effect on the lining of the intestinal tract (see safety information below).

CULINARY USE
Widely available as confectionery, with a pleasant, spicy taste.

SAFETY INFORMATION
Excess licorice can cause fluid retention, headaches, and increased blood pressure; it should not be taken medicinally by people on blood-pressure medication. Licorice should only be used to treat issues such as gastric ulceration under medical supervision.

HAMMAMELIS VIRGINIANA
• WITCH HAZEL

This deciduous shrub produces three or four trunks from a single root and grows up to 16 ft (5 m) in height. Its bark is smooth and gray, and it develops clusters of fragrant yellow flowers in early February or March before the oval leaves form. Originally native to the eastern United States and Canada, witch hazel has been successfully introduced to Europe, where it has naturalized itself easily. The tree needs moderately fertile, well-drained soil in a sunny or partially shady position. If you want to grow witch hazel yourself, it is best sown as seed, first in containers, then by transferring the young plants to the garden. For medicinal use, the twigs are cut just after flowering to make distilled witch hazel water, and the bark is used to make a tincture.

Witch hazel was well known to Native American healers as a potent remedy for ulcers, swellings, bruises, pulled muscles and sore eyes. The plant was given its botanical name "*virginiana*" because it was first collected from the damp woods of Virginia in the USA. The name "witch hazel" is a folk name, possibly linked to the use of young twigs as divining rods in the search for water. Another old name for the tree is "snapping hazelnut" because the seeds are powerfully ejected from their pods when ripe.

SEE ALSO

Arnica, daisy, yarrow, horsetail fern, German camomile

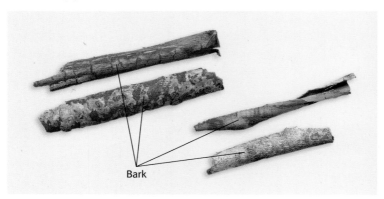

Bark

WITCH HAZEL

Hammamelis virginiana

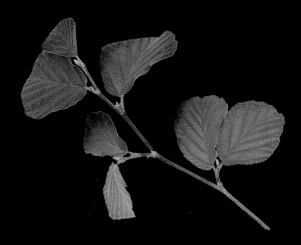

PARTS OF PLANT USED
Leaves, bark, stems

ACTIVE INGREDIENTS
Bitters, glycosides, saponins, tannins

COMMERCIALLY AVAILABLE AS
Tincture, ointment, distilled witch hazel water

ACTIONS
Astringent, anti-inflammatory, antiseptic

USED TO TREAT
Bruises: ointment of witch hazel applied 2–3 times daily helps repair damaged blood vessels just under the skin and reduces swelling.
Varicose veins/hemorrhoids: ointment of witch hazel applied 2–3 times daily has an astringent effect on damaged veins, reducing swelling and shrinking them.
Cuts, wounds, bleeding: distilled witch hazel water can be used straight onto the skin as an antiseptic wash to clean injured parts and stop bleeding.
Pimples, acne, blemishes: ointment or distilled witch hazel water applied to affected areas twice daily heals infection and reduces redness.

CULINARY USE
None

SAFETY INFORMATION
Witch hazel tincture is very strong and should only be used under professional guidance.

HARPOGOPHYTUM PROCUMBENS
• DEVIL'S CLAW

This striking plant has a very stout root that produces secondary storage tubers. Its foliage grows at ground level, with trailing stems and grayish-green leaves. It produces dark red or purple trumpet-shaped flowers and then very distinctive, dramatically spiny fruit, which have given rise to the common name "Devil's claw." It thrives in a sandy, arid environment where it out-competes other plants for water. Devil's claw is native to Africa, specifically to Botswana, Namibia, and South Africa. The side tubers—the active medicinal part—are collected from the wild, as the plant has not yet been successfully cultivated on a commercial scale; Namibia exports around 2,000 tonnes of dried root per year. There are presently conservation concerns about Devil's claw in its native habitat; over-harvesting means that the plant may be under threat.

The medicinal properties of Devil's claw were first analyzed in Germany in the 1950s, when it was shown to contain important anti-inflammatory ingredients. Since then it has been compared to cortisone for its pain-relieving potential. However, only whole extracts containing all the ingredients present in the plant have beneficial effects. It can also be drunk as a tea as a convenient way to absorb its properties.

SEE ALSO

Burdock, wild yam, heather, yellow gentian, calendula

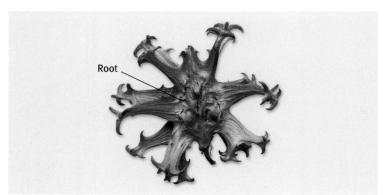

Root

DEVIL'S CLAW

Harpogophytum procumbens

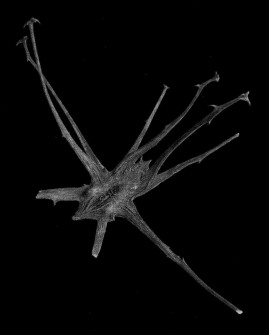

PART OF PLANT USED
Tubers

ACTIVE INGREDIENTS
Beta sitosterols, bitters, gum, iridoid glycosides, resin, sugar

COMMERCIALLY AVAILABLE AS
Capsules, tablets, tincture, tea

ACTIONS
Analgesic, antibacterial, anti-inflammatory, diuretic, laxative, sedative

USED TO TREAT
Arthritis, rheumatism, backache: tablets, capsules, or tincture taken as directed give pain relief and reduce inflammation.
Liver and gallbladder problems: tablets, capsules, or tincture taken as directed stimulate liver and gallbladder function.
Indigestion, heartburn, constipation: tablets, capsules, or tincture taken as directed improve digestive processes and regulate bowel rhythm.
Skin lesions, wounds, boils: the tea, cooled, can be applied to infected or damaged skin 2–3 times daily to disinfect the area and calm inflammation.

CULINARY USE
None

SAFETY INFORMATION
People with diabetes, duodenal or gastric ulcers, high blood pressure or those on cardiac medication should not use Devil's claw. Avoid during pregnancy, as it is a uterine stimulant.

HELIANTHUS ANNUUS
• SUNFLOWER

This very tall annual plant can grow up to 10 ft (3 m), producing large, golden daisy heads, some of which can be as wide as 16 in (40 cm). They have long, bright yellow petals and brown, tubular disc florets in their center where the seeds form. These have black-and-white striped cases, and a single average-sized flower produces approximately 1,000 seeds. Sunflowers thrive in well-drained soil in full sun, but need regular watering in hot weather. Many ornamental varieties exist, with colors ranging from orange to deep reddish-brown, and they are very easy to grow in pots.

The name "*Helianthus*" derives from the Greek words "*helios*" (sun) and "*anthos*" (flower). Sunflowers were originally native to Central America and Mexico, where they were cultivated by indigenous people as far back as 1000 BCE. They were introduced to Europe in the 16th century, but were not grown as a crop until they reached Russia, where large-scale cultivation became extremely successful. Today sunflowers are produced in many countries worldwide; the plants make cattle fodder and the seeds are sold in bulk or pressed to yield a vegetable oil.

SEE ALSO

Gingko, licorice, aloe vera, lavender, evening primrose

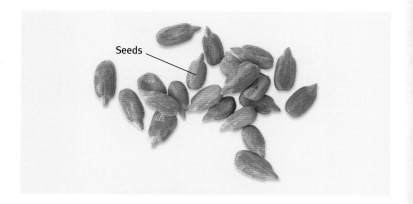

Seeds

SUNFLOWER
Helianthus annuus

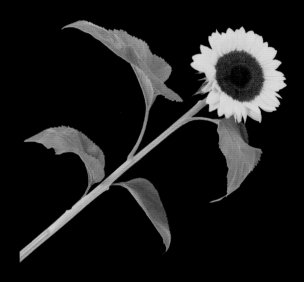

PART OF PLANT USED
Seeds

ACTIVE INGREDIENTS
Inulin, vegetable oil rich in unsaturated linolenic and oleic fatty acids (up to 45 percent) as well as palmitic and arachic acid and vitamin E

COMMERCIALLY AVAILABLE AS
Seeds, vegetable oil

ACTIONS
Anti-asthmatic, skin rejuvenating

USED TO TREAT
Asthma: the inulin content in the seeds and oil has a beneficial effect on the spasms of asthma; included in the diet, both are a useful preventive.

Dry, damaged, or mature skin: sunflower oil makes an excellent massage oil or a base for an ointment or a macerated oil. It is light when applied and does not leave a residue. Its fatty-acid and vitamin-E content make it an excellent skin conditioner.

CULINARY USE
The vegetable oil makes good salad dressings or mayonnaise and is a light cooking oil for frying. The seeds can be toasted and used as salad toppings, or added to bread recipes.

SAFETY INFORMATION
No issues

HIPPOPHAE RHAMNOIDES
• SEA BUCKTHORN

An extremely hardy shrub, sea buckthorn can withstand temperatures from -45°F (-43°C) to 104°F (40°C). It develops an extremely vigorous, sucker-based root system and is therefore ideal for reclaiming land lost to soil erosion and drought. It thrives in all kinds of soils, even the poorest. It is dioecious, meaning that separate plants have male or female flowers, so both sexes need to be grown for fruit production. It is a multi-branched, thorny shrub growing up to 12 ft (4 m) in height. Pale green flowers form on two-year-old wood, before the development of narrow, silver-gray leaves, and the fruit is a small, round, bright orange berry with a very acid taste.

In recent years sea buckthorn has been investigated as a food and medicinal crop with great economic potential. Its fruits, very rich in vitamin C, amino acids, protein, and fatty acids, can be made into beverages and jam. The fatty oil extracted from the fruit has very potent medicinal properties, especially for all kinds of burns, including radiation damage. The leaves and twigs are used to produce an essential oil with skin-healing properties. Sea buckthorn essential oil, fatty oil, leaves, and fruit are used to make many medicinal preparations throughout Asia and Europe.

SEE ALSO
Lavender, aloe vera, evening primrose, borage, lemon

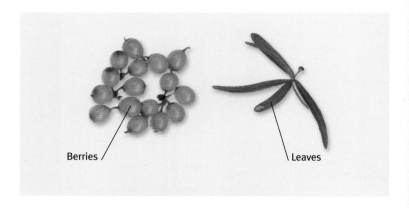

Berries

Leaves

SEA BUCKTHORN

Hippophae rhamnoides

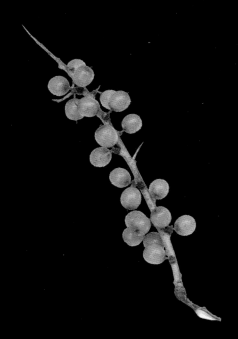

PARTS OF PLANT USED
Leaves, berries

ACTIVE INGREDIENTS
Leaves—tannins, volatile oil; fruits—carbohydrates, protein, fatty acids, amino acids, vitamins C and E

COMMERCIALLY AVAILABLE AS
Capsules (fatty oil), essential oil, tea, jam, juice

ACTIONS
Leaves—astringent; essential oil—anti-inflammatory, skin healing; fruit—immune tonic, stomach tonic

USED TO TREAT
Burns, sunburn, radiation burns: 2 drops of essential oil in 1 teaspoon (5 ml) of sunflower oil applied to affected areas 2–3 times daily relieves pain and inflammation and speeds healing.
Dry, damaged skin: fatty oil of sea buckthorn (split open a capsule and apply to skin) regenerates damaged skin cells and improves skin texture.
Influenza, colds, convalescence, low resistance: sea buckthorn juice or jam taken in the diet is a very high source of protein, amino acids, and vitamin C, and a valuable tonic to the immune system.

CULINARY USE
Jam can be made with sea buckthorn berries.

SAFETY INFORMATION
No issues

HUMULUS LUPUS
• HOP

Originally native to mainland Europe, this perennial climbing herb thrives successfully in hedges and thickets, most often in uncultivated areas. It is now grown commercially all over the world because of its importance in the making of beer. The leaves have three to five lobes and are hairy, and the plant is dioecious. The female flowers, picked and dried, are the medicinally useful part. They are conical in shape, with papery bracts or enlarged petals at their ripest; they have a spicy aroma when they have been dried, due to the presence of a volatile oil.

In Europe, hops have been used to clear, preserve, and flavor beer since the Middle Ages. However, they were not introduced to Britain until the 16th century. Herbal texts of the time mentioned hops' ability to induce melancholy and lower libido, and even maintained they were "dangerous"—most likely because they were a European import in competition with traditional English herbs used to flavor ale. Hops contain sedative ingredients that can help with sleeping problems; they are found in many herbal tea and tablet combinations to improve relaxation.

SEE ALSO

Valerian, melissa, oat, bitter orange, spearmint

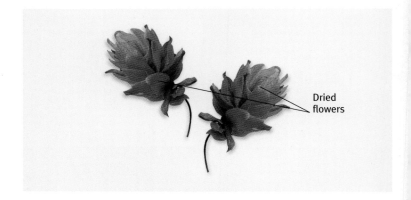

Dried flowers

HOP

Humulus lupus

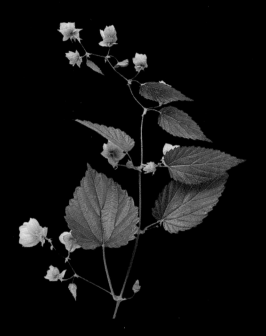

PART OF PLANT USED
Female flowers

ACTIVE INGREDIENTS
Amino acids, bitter resin compound, glycosides, estrogenic compounds, volatile oil

COMMERCIALLY AVAILABLE AS
Tea, tablets, capsules, tincture, herb pillows

ACTIONS
Antispasmodic, digestive tonic, sedative

USED TO TREAT
Insomnia due to emotional stress or an overactive mind: using a hop pillow, drinking tea at night, or taking capsules, tablets, or tincture as directed helps improve the depth and quality of sleep.
Irritability, nervous stress, and tension: hops have a restorative effect on the nervous system, taken in the above preparations or used as a hop pillow.
Indigestion of nervous origin: tea taken after meals settles the digestion and has a relaxing effect on emotional stress.

CULINARY USE
Beer making

SAFETY INFORMATION
Large doses can disrupt the menstrual cycle; always follow manufacturers' guidelines. Best avoided in pregnancy because of the hormonal effect, also by those with estrogen-dependent cancers. People with depression should not use hops because of the sedative effect.

HYDRASTIS CANADENSIS
• GOLDENSEAL

This woodland plant is native to the United States, specifically to Ohio, Indiana, West Virginia, Kentucky, and parts of Illinois. Over-harvesting has led to depletion in its native habitat, so goldenseal is now cultivated commercially in Washington State and North Carolina. It is a low-growing member of the buttercup family. The roots form twisted, knotted, yellow clumps, its stems are hairy, and its leaves have a wrinkled appearance. It produces white flowers in the spring. The roots are the active medicinal part, also yielding a yellow dye—they are harvested after at least two years' growth and dried before being processed.

Goldenseal is one of many herbs that were adopted by early settlers to the United States, following the medicinal practice of Native American healers. The Cherokee, Iroquois, Catawba, and Kickapoo tribes used goldenseal in various ways, for example, as an antiseptic, a wash for sore eyes, an insect repellent, a digestive remedy, and an immune tonic. It was mentioned in the notes of Captain Lewis in 1804, on the Lewis and Clark expedition to the Pacific coast, as being an excellent remedy for eye troubles and sore mouths. Today, one of the main alkaloid ingredients of goldenseal—berberine—is being investigated for potential antiviral effects.

SEE ALSO
Eyebright, cornflower, echinacea, myrrh, dill

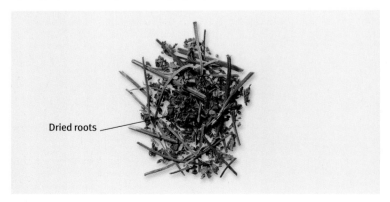

Dried roots

GOLDENSEAL
Hydrastis canadensis

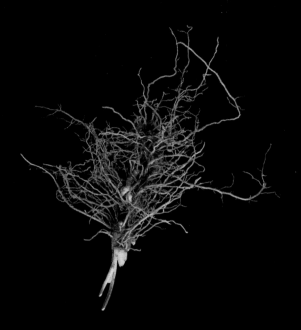

PART OF PLANT USED
Roots

ACTIVE INGREDIENTS
Alkaloids, resin, volatile oil

COMMERCIALLY AVAILABLE AS
Tablets, capsules, tincture, eye drops

ACTIONS
Antiseptic, digestive tonic, expectorant, laxative, immune tonic

USED TO TREAT
Catarrh, bronchitis: tablets, capsules, or tincture taken as directed help to clear chronic catarrh and infection.
Sore, inflamed eyes, minor eye infections: infusion of the roots, cooled, applied twice daily, or eye drops used as directed will heal infections associated with the eyes.
Infected gums, sore throats: a dose of tincture in water as directed, used 2–3 times daily as a mouthwash or gargle, clears infection.
Constipation, sluggish digestion: tablets, capsules, or tincture taken as directed stimulate bowel rhythm and improve digestion.

CULINARY USE
None

SAFETY INFORMATION
Do not use in pregnancy as it is a uterine stimulant. People under medical care for cardiovascular problems should seek medical advice before using goldenseal because of its high alkaloid content.

HYPERICUM PERFORATUM
• ST. JOHN'S WORT

This hardy perennial herb grows up to 2 ft (60 cm) in height, with erect, partly woody stems and opposite pairs of oval leaves speckled with tiny oil glands (hence the Latin name "*perforatum*" or perforated). The golden yellow flowers have five petals. St. John's wort grows best in well-drained, lime-rich soil, in sun or partial shade, and spreads rapidly once established. Its natural habitat is along river banks, hedgerows or in woodland. In cultivation, it is best propagated by dividing root clumps and replanting. Many ornamental varieties exist; however, this species is the one required for medicinal use. The flowering stems need to be picked from July onwards; they can be dried, or fresh flowers can be soaked in oil (macerated) to produce an herbal oil (see page 298), which will turn red thanks to the main ingredient, hypericin.

142

The name "*Hypericum*" is derived from a Greek phrase meaning "over an apparition." Since ancient times, this herb has been considered to have strong protective powers against the supernatural, and in medieval times it was hung in doorways and windows to repel evil spirits. In the Middle Ages the knights of St. John used it extensively to heal sword wounds among the crusaders, hence the first part of the common name.

SEE ALSO
Aloe vera, lavender, sea buckthorn, melissa, clary sage

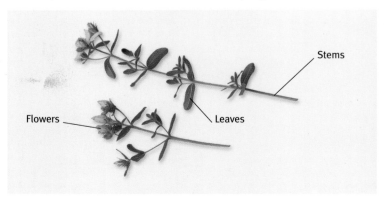

Stems

Flowers

Leaves

ST. JOHN'S WORT

Hypericum perforatum

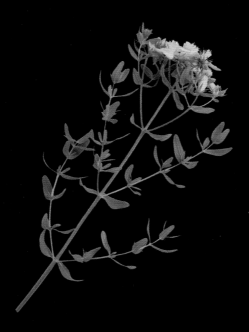

PART OF PLANT USED
Flowering tops

ACTIVE INGREDIENTS
Flavonoid glycosides (including red pigmented hypericin), tannins, volatile oil

COMMERCIALLY AVAILABLE AS
Tablets, capsules, tincture, macerated oil

ACTIONS
Anti-inflammatory, antiseptic, astringent, sedative

USED TO TREAT
Burns, wounds, bruises, deep cuts: macerated oil applied 2–3 times daily to affected areas heals skin, reduces inflammation and clears infection.
Neuralgia, sciatica: macerated oil applied 2–3 times daily to affected areas has a pain-relieving effect.
Depression, mood swings, menopausal emotional tension: tablets, capsules, or tincture taken as directed help to calm mental and emotional stress.
Menstrual cramps: macerated oil applied 2–3 times daily to the abdomen eases menstrual pain.

CULINARY USE
None

SAFETY INFORMATION
Prolonged use of the herb may make some people hypersensitive to sunlight. Anyone on antidepressant medication should check with a doctor before using this herb. St. John's wort is contraindicated for the contraceptive pill.

HYSSOPUS OFFICINALIS
• HYSSOP

This hardy, aromatic herb is a member of the same plant family as lavender and rosemary. It is considered semi-evergreen because it can withstand winter temperatures, although it does lose leaves in heavy frosts. It grows up to 3 ft (1 m) in height with woody stems at the base, small, scented, dark green foliage, and spikes of deep purple-blue flowers from June to August. It is very attractive to bees and butterflies. Originally native to the Mediterranean, it thrives in full sun, hot temperatures, and dry, stony soil. It can be grown from seed or from softwood cuttings taken from a parent plant in summer. Bushes need hard pruning in early spring to prevent them becoming straggly. The flowering tops are used medicinally, either dried, made into tincture, or distilled to produce an essential oil.

The ancient Greek physician Dioscorides in the 1st century CE called this plant "*Hyssopus*" from the Hebrew "*esob*," meaning "holy herb." However, modern herbalists believe that it is unlikely that this plant is the hyssop of the Bible. Dioscorides valued this plant for the treatment of respiratory complaints, and in the 17th century the English herbalist Nicholas Culpeper recommended making hyssop syrup to ease bad coughs or chest infections. It is still a key ingredient in commercial herbal cough mixtures to this day.

SEE ALSO

White horehound, goldenseal, heather, centaury, tea tree

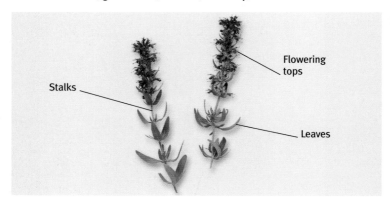

Flowering tops

Stalks

Leaves

HYSSOP

Hyssopus officinalis

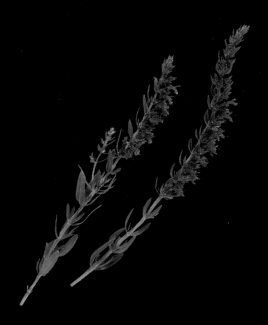

PART OF PLANT USED
Flowering tops

ACTIVE INGREDIENTS
Bitters, glycosides, tannins, volatile oil
with pinocamphone

COMMERCIALLY AVAILABLE AS
Essential oil, tincture, herbal
cough mixtures

ACTIONS
Anti-inflammatory, astringent, diuretic,
emmenagogue, expectorant

USED TO TREAT
*Stubborn coughs, bronchitis, chest
infections:* herbal cough mixture taken
as directed soothes irritated bronchial
passages and stops irritated spasmodic
coughing, as well as helping get rid
of excess mucus.
Rheumatism: a hot bath with 2 handfuls
of fresh flowers added to it is an old folk
remedy for rheumatic pain and stiffness.
Insect bites and stings: infusion of fresh
flowers, cooled and applied to bites
and stings relieves pain and reduces
swelling; or 20 drops of tincture in 3 fl oz
(100 ml) of water can be applied for the
same effect.

CULINARY USE
None

SAFETY INFORMATION
Hyssop should never be used by
epileptics, nor in pregnancy, because it
stimulates menstruation.

JUNIPERUS COMMUNIS
• JUNIPER

A tough, coniferous, evergreen shrub, juniper can grow up to 13 ft(4 m) in height. It has reddish-brown twigs and blue-green needles. The berries are borne on female plants and stay green for more than two years before they ripen and turn blue-black, when they are ready to be harvested. Juniper needs a sunny position and will tolerate most soils, though it thrives best in lime-rich ground. Native all over northern Europe, it grows naturally on the edges of woods or heathland, and requires a lot of moisture. It can be grown from seed or from cuttings taken in spring; once bushes take they spread vigorously.

For hundreds of years, juniper berries have been used as a protective remedy against all manner of toxins, such as poisons, snakebites, and even bubonic plague—in the Middle Ages, twigs and branches were burned in sick rooms to purify the air. The name "juniper" is a corruption of the Dutch word "*genever*," the original name for gin, the alcoholic drink flavored with ripe juniper berries. In Germany and Switzerland a jam made with ripe berries is still traditionally eaten in the winter to prevent colds and influenza.

SEE ALSO

Angelica, Devil's claw, rosemary, black pepper, bearberry/uva ursi

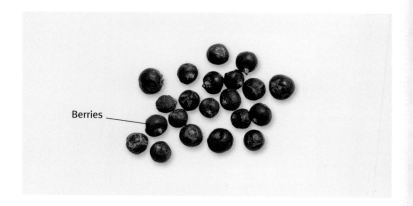

Berries

JUNIPER

Juniperus communis

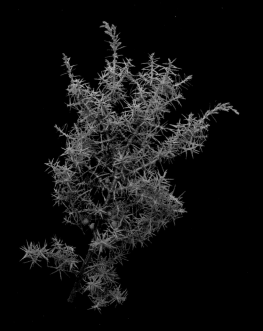

PART OF PLANT USED
Berries

ACTIVE INGREDIENTS
Flavinoids, resin, sugar, tannins, vitamin C, volatile oil

COMMERCIALLY AVAILABLE AS
Dried berries, essential oil, tincture, massage balm

ACTIONS
Antiseptic, diuretic, local circulation stimulant, carminative

USED TO TREAT
Rheumatism, gout, osteoarthritis: massage balm applied 2–3 times daily to affected parts eases pain and stimulates tissue detoxification.

Muscular aches and pains, poor circulation: 4 drops of essential oil in 2 teaspoons (10 ml) of sunflower oil massaged into affected areas warms the muscles and eases pain or stiffness.
Fluid retention: tincture taken as directed stimulates the kidneys.

CULINARY USE
In northern Europe juniper berries are cooked with red cabbage and apple, or with "*sauerkraut*" (salted cabbage).

SAFETY INFORMATION
Anyone with kidney disease should not use juniper remedies internally. Use of juniper preparations for more than six weeks is not recommended because it is a strong diuretic. Avoid during pregnancy because of the stimulating effects.

LAURUS NOBILIS
• BAY LAUREL

Bay trees are evergreen and very aromatic, with lance-shaped, olive-green leaves and small, yellow flowers. If they are planted in the ground they can grow to 50 ft (15 m) in height, so drastic pruning of lead branches to prevent height and spread is needed in a small garden. A popular style is to clip the tree into a spherical crown. Bay trees also thrive in pots, provided they are given moderately rich soil and a sunny location. Originally native to southern Europe and North Africa, bay trees thrive in intense heat; in cooler climates they need protection from frost and cold winds in the winter. The leaves—the important aromatic and medicinal part of the tree—are best gathered for drying in high summer, when the volatile-oil content is highest. However, fresh leaves can be used all year round.

The Romans made extensive use of bay leaves—they were used to make the original "laurel wreaths" worn by generals celebrating victories, as well as being made into garlands and sacred offerings. Bay trees were introduced to Britain in the 16th century and became popular in designs for European-influenced, geometrically perfect "parterre" gardens in stately homes.

SEE ALSO

Cardamom, ginger, rosemary, peppermint, fennel

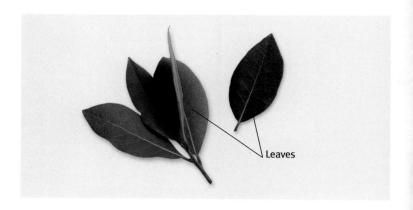

Leaves

BAY LAUREL

Laurus nobilis

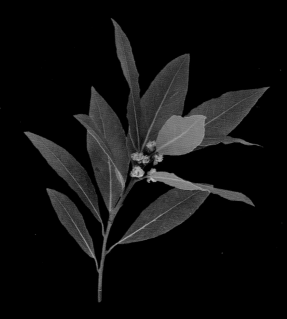

PART OF PLANT USED
Leaves

ACTIVE INGREDIENTS
Bitters, tannins, volatile oil

COMMERCIALLY AVAILABLE AS
Dried leaves, essential oil

ACTIONS
Antimicrobial, carminative, digestive tonic, immune tonic, local circulation stimulant

USED TO TREAT
Colds, influenza: 2 drops of essential oil in a warm bathtub eases chills and aches, and improves breathing.
Muscular aches and pains: 4 drops of essential oil in 2 teaspoons (10 ml) of sunflower oil massaged into affected areas twice daily warms the circulation and eases stiffness.
Indigestion: bay leaves used in cooking, as well as two drops of essential oil in 1 teaspoon (5 ml) of sunflower oil massaged into the abdomen twice daily, eases gas and digestive cramps.

CULINARY USE
Bay leaves are commonly used as a flavoring for meat or vegetable stews, soups, fish dishes, Bolognese sauce, and also sometimes as a flavoring in milk puddings. The leaves release their aroma more effectively if a dish is simmered slowly for a long time.

SAFETY INFORMATION
No issues

LAVENDULA ANGUSTIFOLIA
• LAVENDER

At least 80 species and countless varieties of lavender are now grown all over the world. *Lavandula angustifolia* is the most common species, grown commercially to produce essential oil. Lavender is an aromatic shrub growing up to 3 ft (1 m) in height, with compact, woody stems at the base and gray-green foliage. It produces tall spikes of tiny, purple flowers in midsummer. It needs full sun, and light, sandy soil to produce the best aroma. Bushes need pruning back hard in late summer or early spring to keep them in shape. Taking cuttings from parent plants in late spring is the best way to propagate lavender. For medicinal use, flowering tops should be harvested just before they are in full bloom, usually around the end of July, and the stalks hung upside down in a warm place to dry.

Lavender is originally native to the southern Mediterranean, and was probably brought to Britain by the Romans (the name "lavender" comes from the Latin "*lavare*," meaning "to wash"). It was a popular plant in the gardens of the poor, and also featured in aromatic hedges and formal layouts in stately homes. Today lavender essential oil is one of the most popular aromatherapy oils, to help stress-related problems and insomnia.

SEE ALSO
Aloe vera, yarrow, pasque flower, rosemary, valerian

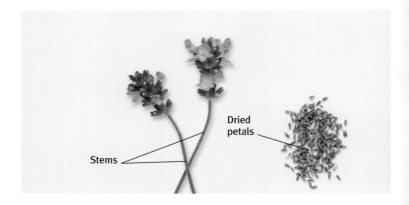

Dried petals

Stems

LAVENDER

Lavendula angustifolia

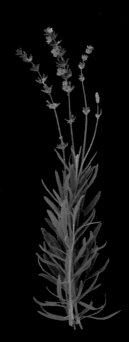

PART OF PLANT USED
Flowering tops

ACTIVE INGREDIENTS
Tannins, volatile oil

COMMERCIALLY AVAILABLE AS
Dried flowers, essential oil, massage balm, ointment, gargle

ACTIONS
Analgesic, antiseptic, antispasmodic, sedative, vulnerary

USED TO TREAT
Burns, wounds, damaged skin, pimples, insect bites, and stings: 2 drops of neat essential oil on a cotton pad applied directly to damaged areas 2–3 times daily disinfects skin and speeds healing.

Headaches, migraine, PMS: 2 drops of neat essential oil rubbed onto the forehead and temples as needed soothes pain.
Muscular aches and pains: massage balm or ointment or 4 drops of essential oil in 2 teaspoons (10 ml) of sunflower oil applied to affected areas twice daily eases pain and stiffness.
Insomnia: 2 drops of neat essential oil on the pillow helps calm the mind and improves relaxation.

CULINARY USE
Dried lavender flowers can be added to scones or ice cream.

SAFETY INFORMATION
No issues

LEONURUS CARDIACA
• MOTHERWORT

A perennial herb that grows up to 3 ft (1 m) in height, motherwort produces an erect, tough, four-sided stem. Its leaves are in opposing pairs; they have three to five lobes, and are a vivid green on the upper surface and pale and hairy beneath, with serrated edges. The flowers are produced in the axils of the leaves, where the leaf stems join the main stem, and are small and pinkish-white in color. The whole plant has a rather unpleasant odor but is very attractive to bees. It can easily be grown from seed and will self-seed once established. It prefers a sunny location. Motherwort was originally native to Siberia but has naturalized itself all over Europe. The flowering stems are the medicinally active part of the plant, and these need to be harvested in August when the plant is in full bloom, and then dried carefully.

As the name suggests, motherwort or "mother herb" has been traditionally used for centuries to help women in childbirth and those with menopausal problems, such as nervous tension. Old herbal texts praise it as an herb to strengthen the heart and combat fear, which is what it was intended to do during labor. Today, the herb is used more for its sedative properties.

SEE ALSO

Lavender, valerian, melissa, black cohosh, sage

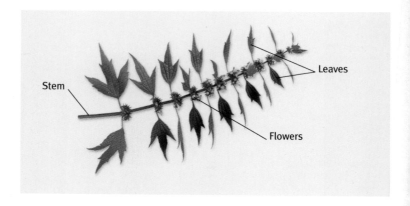

Stem

Leaves

Flowers

MOTHERWORT

Leonurus cardiaca

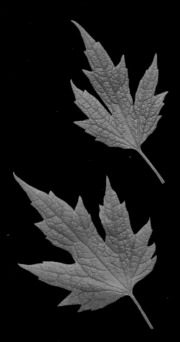

PART OF PLANT USED
Flowering tops

ACTIVE INGREDIENTS
Alkaloids, bitters, glycosides, tannins, volatile oil

COMMERCIALLY AVAILABLE AS
Tablets, tincture

ACTIONS
Antispasmodic, cardiotonic, hypotensive, sedative

USED TO TREAT
Insomnia, especially stress-related: tablets or tincture taken as directed have a sedative effect on the mind, improving relaxation and sleep.
Migraines, headaches, including PMS-related headaches: tablets or tincture taken as directed ease spasmodic pain.
Menopausal issues (low energy, tiredness): tablets or tincture taken as directed help to ease stress and emotional tension.
High blood pressure: tablets or tincture taken as directed have a hypotensive effect, lowering blood pressure.

CULINARY USE
None

SAFETY INFORMATION
Anyone on cardiac medication or medically diagnosed with high blood pressure should consult a doctor or medical herbalist before using the herb. Do not use in pregnancy, as it is a uterine tonic.

LEPTOSPERMUM SCOPARIUM
• MANUKA

Native throughout New Zealand, manuka bushes are highly aromatic; they belong to the same plant family as tea tree (see pages 166–7) and eucalyptus (see pages 108–9). They are very vigorous and spread by self-seeding. Shrubs are typically about 12 ft (4 m) tall. Manuka has small, hairy, lance-shaped leaves and white or pinkish flowers from September to February. The leaves are filled with sacs containing a powerful volatile oil, giving the whole plant a pungent aroma.

The Maori valued manuka as a healing herb, calling it "*kahikatoa*" or "*pata*." They made steam inhalations of leaves in boiling water to help respiratory problems, or crushed seed capsules into a pulp to dress wounds. Today, it is an important commercial source of essential oil and honey, which has been analyzed and shown to contain special enzymes with dramatic antibacterial effects. Many hospitals in New Zealand now use manuka-honey dressings to treat burns, skin ulcers, and infected wounds, with speedy results. The quality of manuka honey varies according to the amount of healing enzymes it contains; this is shown numerically, with potencies of 4 or 5 being low, and 10 and above having higher antibacterial activity.

SEE ALSO

Myrrh, tea tree, eucalyptus, black pepper, white horehound

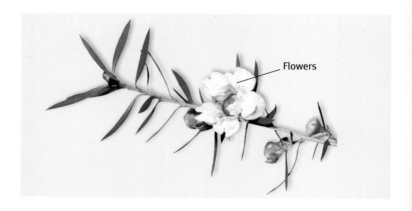

Flowers

MANUKA

Leptospermum scoparium

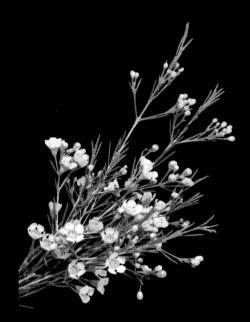

PARTS OF PLANT USED
Flowers, leaves

ACTIVE INGREDIENTS
Flowers — enzymes; volatile oil —
terpenes, triketones

COMMERCIALLY AVAILABLE AS
Honey, essential oil

ACTIONS
Honey — antibacterial, vulnerary;
essential oil — expectorant, antiseptic,
immune stimulant

USED TO TREAT
Wounds, ulcers, skin infections: 1 or
2 teaspoons (5–10 ml) of honey can
be applied directly 2–3 times daily, to
cleanse the area and speed healing.

Colds, influenza: 1 teaspoon (5 ml) of
honey can be taken in 10 fl oz (300 ml)
of hot water with a slice of lemon as an
immune-boosting drink, 3–4 times daily;
add 3 drops of essential oil to 10 fl oz
(300 ml) of boiling water and inhale the
steam for 10 minutes to ease breathing.
Coughs: 2 drops of essential oil in 1
teaspoon (5 ml) of sunflower oil can be
massaged into the chest twice daily to
ease coughing and help breathing.

CULINARY USE
Honey can be eaten in the diet as a
preventive, immune-boosting food
supplement in the winter.

SAFETY INFORMATION
No issues

LEVISTICUM OFFICINALE
• LOVAGE

This very hardy, herbaceous perennial herb has deep, fleshy roots, and stems up to 6 ft (3 m) tall. Its glossy green leaves have a spicy aroma and it produces umbels of yellowish flowers in July and August, followed by small seeds. It likes moist soil in sun or partial shade and needs plenty of nutrients. Although it can be grown from seed, it is best propagated in the fall by dividing roots into two or three clumps and replanting them separately. Leaves can be harvested fresh throughout spring and summer. Roots should be at least three years old before harvesting for medicinal use.

Lovage is an old English cottage-garden herb, which was valued for centuries as a seasoning, a digestive tonic, and even an aphrodisiac—the name "lovage" is from the old English "love-ache." The English 17th-century herbalist Nicholas Culpeper used it for digestive cramps, easing gas, and producing sweating; he regarded it as a stimulating and warming herb. In old-fashioned country recipes crushed lovage seeds were used like pepper to flavor dishes, because of their hot taste; they were also used in the bathtub as a warming treatment for rheumatism.

SEE ALSO
Elder, yarrow, fennel, yellow gentian, heather

Dried roots

LOVAGE

Levisticum officinale

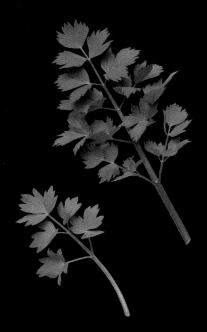

PART OF PLANT USED
Dried roots, seeds

ACTIVE INGREDIENTS
Coumarins, esters, resin, volatile oil

COMMERCIALLY AVAILABLE AS
Dried roots, dried seeds, essential oil

ACTIONS
Digestive tonic, diuretic, expectorant,
liver tonic

USED TO TREAT
Influenza: infusion of dried root taken
2–3 times daily promotes sweating and
helps support the body through the
course of a viral infection.
Sluggish digestion, indigestion, gas:
half a teaspoon (2.5 g) of dried seeds,
chewed after a meal, settles the
digestion and stimulates the liver.
Rheumatism: 1 tablespoon (20 g) of
dried seeds, crushed and placed in
a muslin bag, then soaked in a hot
bathtub, eases pain and stiffness.

CULINARY USE
Young lovage leaves can be added to
salad combinations or made into
soup, and the seeds can be added to
bread dough.

SAFETY INFORMATION
Avoid lovage in pregnancy as it can
stimulate menstruation. Because of the
strong diuretic effect, avoid it in cases of
kidney or bladder disease. The essential
oil is phototoxic; avoid direct skin
exposure to UV rays after application.

LIPPIA CITRIODORA
• LEMON VERBENA

This attractive, deciduous shrub grows up to 15 ft (5 m) tall. It has strongly lemon-scented pointed leaves, 3–4 in (7–10 cm) long, dotted underneath with sacs containing volatile oil. In hot climates, spikes of tiny, pinkish-white flowers appear in late summer. In cooler latitudes it will not flower. It can survive at temperatures as low as 23°F (–5°C) but must have shelter and be exposed to strong sunlight in the daytime. If persistent frosts are a problem, try planting it in a pot and bringing it into a conservatory or greenhouse during the winter. Lemon verbena shrubs need hard pruning in spring and can be propagated from cuttings. The leaves can be harvested throughout the summer and used fresh for making tea, or dried for storage (after many months they still retain their pleasant lemon-scented aroma).

This shrub is originally native to South America, particularly Peru and the Andes, where the leaves are still used extensively to make teas, as well as many natural cosmetics and toiletries. Verbena was introduced to Europe in the late 18th century and spread throughout the continent, becoming popular in Victorian times in dried herb sachets, herb pillows, and perfume formulae. In France it has become one of the most popular herbal teas, "*verveine*," served in cafés and restaurants as a digestive tonic after meals.

SEE ALSO

Ginger, peppermint, fennel, lavender, melissa

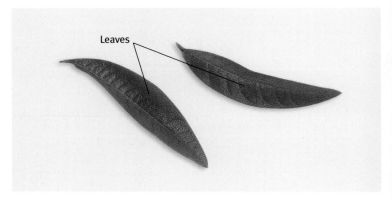

Leaves

LEMON VERBENA

Lippia citriodora

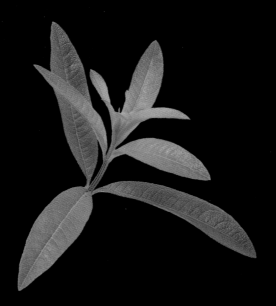

PART OF PLANT USED
Leaves

ACTIVE INGREDIENTS
Volatile oil

COMMERCIALLY AVAILABLE AS
Tea

ACTIONS
Antispasmodic, carminative,
digestive tonic

USED TO TREAT
Digestive nausea: tea taken 2–3 times
daily eases waves of sickness and calms
the stomach.
Indigestion, gas: tea taken after meals
stimulates the digestion and releases
gas in the bowel.

Digestive migraine: lemon verbena tea
taken 2–3 times daily eases headaches
caused by food allergies.
Insomnia due to emotional stress: tea
taken in the evening before bed calms
anxiety and aids relaxation.

CULINARY USE
Try one or two few fresh lemon verbena
leaves, chopped finely, to add an
unusual lemon flavor to green-leaf
salad combinations.

SAFETY INFORMATION
No issues

LOBELIA INFLATA
• LOBELIA

As its other common name "Indian tobacco" suggests, this is a North American plant, originally smoked by Native Americans as an alternative to tobacco, and used in native medicine as a relaxing remedy. It is an annual plant, growing up to 2 ft (60 cm) in height; its leaves are lance-shaped with a serrated edge. Its flowers are pale blue-violet in color with yellow centers, and the seeds are brown. It is native to Massachusetts, Georgia, Kansas, Arkansas, and parts of Canada, where it thrives in meadows, fields, by roads, in woods, or on waste ground, usually in dry soil. Lobelia can be obtained in horticultural varieties with scarlet, purple, or blue flowers, but none of these are medicinally potent. Flowering tops of _Lobelia inflata_ are harvested in summer and the herb can be used fresh or dried to preserve the active ingredients.

Today, lobelia is restricted to professional herbalists, who prescribe it as a relaxant, or for asthma or severe respiratory disorders, such as chronic bronchitis. An alkaloid ingredient first identified in 1838, named "lobeline," has powerful effects on the nervous and respiratory systems, making this herb too strong to be made available over the counter to the general public. It needs to be used under professional guidance.

SEE ALSO
Ginkgo, licorice, myrrh, cardamom, rosemary

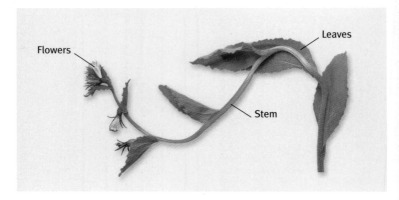

Flowers

Leaves

Stem

LOBELIA
Lobelia inflata

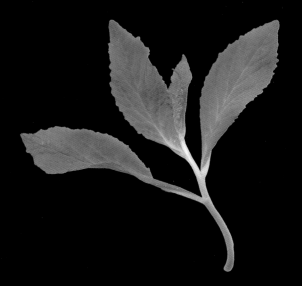

PART OF PLANT USED
Flowering tops

ACTIVE INGREDIENTS
Alkaloids, glycosides, gum, resin, volatile oil

COMMERCIALLY AVAILABLE AS
Restricted to professional herbalists only

ACTIONS
Antispasmodic, respiratory relaxant, narcotic

USED TO TREAT
Professional herbalists prescribe lobelia to treat asthma, chronic bronchitis, and persistent respiratory problems, and as a remedy to help relax the central nervous system. Its use by Native Americans as an alternative to tobacco has led to it being tried as a natural treatment to help people quit smoking. Externally, professionals sometimes use lobelia plasters and poultices to ease sprains, whiplash, torn muscles, and bruises.

CULINARY USE
None

SAFETY INFORMATION
Lobelia must only be used under professional guidance, especially if medication is already being taken for asthma or other respiratory conditions. In excess lobelia can cause vomiting or drowsiness.

MARRUBIUM VULGARE
• WHITE HOREHOUND

This perennial herb grows from a stubby root, producing four-sided stems and wrinkled, toothed, hairy, pointed leaves. In summertime clusters of tiny, white flowers appear in the joints between the leaves and the stems. The whole plant has a very pleasant apple-like smell. White horehound is easy to grow in an herb garden, tolerating most soil types, even poor. It can be sown from seed in spring, or cuttings can be taken from older plants, or root clumps can be divided in the fall and replanted. White horehound does not flower until it is two years old. The flowers, stalks, and leaves are harvested in late summer and can be used fresh, or dried and stored.

Horehound has been used medicinally since Roman times. Its botanical name "*Marrubium*" derives from the Hebrew "*marrob*," the name of a particularly bitter herb used by Jews during the Passover feast. White horehound was well known in northern Europe by the 16th century, when the English herbalist John Gerard mentioned the effectiveness of horehound syrup for coughs, wheezing, and shortness of breath. "Horehound candy" was a popular herbal lozenge in the 19th and early 20th centuries to soothe coughing. The herb is still widely used today, either on its own or in combination with other expectorant herbs to make herbal cough mixture, suitable for both adults and children.

SEE ALSO
Goldenseal, daisy, yellow gentian, cornflower, clary sage

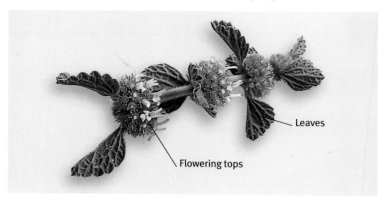

Leaves

Flowering tops

WHITE HOREHOUND

Marrubium vulgare

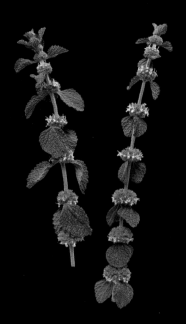

PART OF PLANT USED
Flowering tops

ACTIVE INGREDIENTS
Alcohols, alkaloids, bitters, resin,
saponins, tannins

COMMERCIALLY AVAILABLE AS
Cough mixture, tablets, tincture

ACTIONS
Antispasmodic, emmenagogue,
expectorant, sedative

USED TO TREAT
*Coughs—especially spasmodic with
a lot of phlegm:* cough mixture taken
as directed calms irritated spasms and
helps loosen phlegm and catarrh.
Wounds, cuts, skin inflammation: an
infusion of fresh leaves, cooled, cleans
and disinfects damaged areas.
Liver and gallbladder problems: tablets
or tincture taken as directed stimulate
liver and gallbladder function due to the
bitters in the herb.
Irregular menstruation/PMS: tablets
or tincture taken as directed help to
balance irregular menstrual cycles
and ease PMS symptoms, such as
mood swings.

CULINARY USE
None

SAFETY INFORMATION
Do not use in pregnancy because it
stimulates menstruation.

MATRICARIA CHAMOMILLA
• GERMAN CAMOMILE

German camomile is an annual herb growing up to 2 ft (60 cm) in height with feathery aromatic leaves and solitary flower heads at the end of branching stalks. These have raised golden centers surrounded by white petals. Its other common name is "scented mayweed," giving a clue as to its flowering time—late spring. German camomile is easy to grow from seed in a garden, and it is cultivated on a commercial scale in Germany and central Europe. The scent of the whole plant is stronger and more bitter than Roman camomile (see page 40) thanks to pungent ingredients including volatile oil. Via distillation it yields a dark blue essential oil rich in a constituent called "azulene," which is strongly anti-inflammatory.

The name "camomile" comes from the Greek "*kamai melon*" which literally means "ground apple" (the herb is low-growing with an apple-like aroma).

The strongly aromatic flowers were strewn over floors in medieval times to scent rooms. In the 17th century the English herbalist Nicholas Culpeper called German camomile the "plants' physician," because the plant helps promote the general health of a garden by attracting beneficial insects that naturally feed on pests. Eternally popular in herbal medicine to this day, this is the species of camomile that is most commonly sold as tea.

SEE ALSO
Roman camomile, yarrow, red clover, St. John's wort, Devil's claw

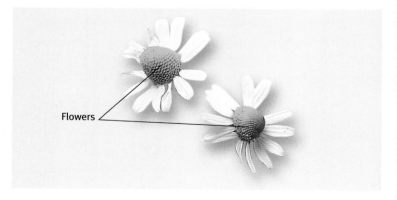

Flowers

GERMAN CAMOMILE

Matricaria chamomilla

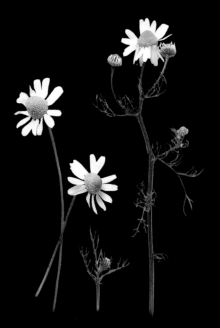

PART OF PLANT USED
Flowers

ACTIVE INGREDIENTS
Fatty acids, flavonoid glycosides, mucilage, volatile oil

COMMERCIALLY AVAILABLE AS
Essential oil, tea, ointment, tablets

ACTIONS
Anti-inflammatory, antispasmodic, sedative, vulnerary

USED TO TREAT
Skin irritation, nappy rash, nettlerash, hives, eczema, sunburn: 2 drops of essential oil in 1 teaspoon (5 ml) of sunflower oil applied to affected areas 2–3 times daily soothes itching and calms redness; camomile ointment can be applied in the same way.
Insomnia, mood swings, irritability: tea taken 2–3 times daily, especially at night, soothes bad moods and calms emotional stress.
Indigestion, stomach cramps: tea or tablets taken as directed ease cramping pains and improve digestive rhythm.
Liver and gall-bladder problems: tea or tablets taken as directed stimulate liver and gall-bladder function, helping digestion of fatty foods.

CULINARY USE
None

SAFETY INFORMATION
No issues

MELALEUCA ALTERNIFOLIA
• TEA TREE

Tea-tree essential oil is now known all over the world as a powerful natural antiseptic. It comes from an evergreen tree native to Australia, a member of the botanical family that includes eucalyptus (see pages 108–9) and manuka (see pages 154–5). Tea tree grows up to 20 ft (7 m) in height with narrow, needle-like leaves, and papery bark which peels off regularly. It produces small, yellow flowers. The volatile oil in the leaves gives the tree a strong aroma, and these are picked and distilled to produce tea-tree essential oil. This is now produced on a massive commercial scale in New South Wales, Australia, though tea tree still grows wild in many other areas.

The Australian Aborigines were well aware of tea tree's healing effects; they made inhalations with the leaves in boiling water to help coughs, chewed the leaves to disinfect the mouth, and made a paste with them to heal wounds. The name "tea tree" was given to the species by sailors on Captain Cook's voyage to Australia in the 18th century because they drank an infusion of the leaves. Tea tree first attracted wide scale attention in World War I when it was used as a wound-cleansing agent.

SEE ALSO

Myrrh, witch hazel, garlic, goldenseal, echinacea

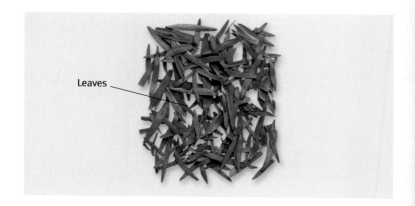

Leaves

TEA TREE

Melaleuca alternifolia

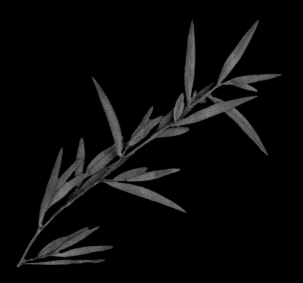

PART OF PLANT USED
Leaves

ACTIVE INGREDIENTS
Volatile oil

COMMERCIALLY AVAILABLE AS
Essential oil, ointment, toothpaste,
mouthwash, shampoo, toiletries,
face cream

ACTIONS
Antiseptic, antimicrobial, antiviral,
vulnerary

USED TO TREAT
Wounds, cuts: 2 drops of essential oil
in a bowl of warm water makes a simple
wound-cleansing solution.
Boils, acne: 2 drops of essential oil neat
on a cotton bud applied to affected areas
2–3 times daily combats infection and
heals blemishes.
Yeast infections, athlete's foot: 2 drops
of essential oil in a warm bathtub helps
soothe and combat infection.
*Sore throats, mouth infections, sore
gums:* mouthwash used twice daily
clears infection and soothes sore tissue.
Influenza, coughs, respiratory infections:
2 drops of essential oil in a warm bathtub
at night helps breathing.

CULINARY USE
None

SAFETY INFORMATION
Do not apply essential oil to sensitive,
damaged, or allergy-prone skin, or to
children under the age of five.

MELISSA OFFICINALIS
• MELISSA

This vigorous perennial herb dies back each year and produces new spring shoots from its base, growing up to 3 ft (1 m) in height, with tough, four-sided stems and strongly lemon-scented, rough-textured, toothed leaves. It grows in most soils, preferring sun or partial shade. It self-seeds easily once established, meaning it spreads quickly, so in an herb garden it may need containing in pots. Melissa produces tiny white flowers in July and August; to maximize leaf production for tea making, pinch out the flowers and more leaves will form. Melissa wilts quickly and loses its fragrance when picked, so it is best used fresh, though it is dried for use in commercially available herbal tea blends.

The name "*Melissa*" comes from the Greek word for bee, and the honey from bees feeding on the flowers is delicious. "Sweet balm" or "bee balm" are other common names for the plant, which attracts many beneficial insects to a garden. Medicinally, melissa has been used for centuries as a wound healer and also to calm and soothe the nerves. Melissa leaves steeped in wine were a popular 19th-century tonic for depression and mental stress. Today it features in herbal tablet combinations for indigestion and insomnia.

SEE ALSO
Roman camomile, yarrow, eyebright, valerian, spearmint

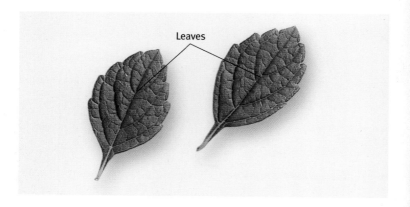

Leaves

MELISSA
Melissa officinalis

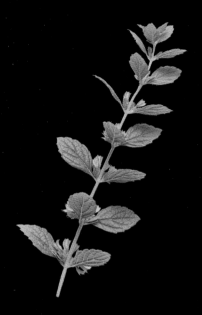

PART OF PLANT USED
Leaves

ACTIVE INGREDIENTS
Flavonoids, tannins, volatile oil

COMMERCIALLY AVAILABLE AS
Essential oil, tea, tablets

ACTIONS
Antiseptic, antihistamine,
antispasmodic, sedative

USED TO TREAT
Nettle rash, insect bites and stings:
infusion of fresh leaves, cooled, then
applied to affected parts as needed
calms itching and reduces inflammation.
Hay fever: tea drunk 3–4 times daily has
a mild antihistamine effect.

Insomnia, mental stress: tea drunk
before bed helps to calm and relax
the mind.
Indigestion: tea taken after meals settles
the stomach and calms spasms.
Cold sores, chicken pox, shingles: 2
drops of essential oil (it is rare and
expensive) added to 1 teaspoon (5 ml)
of sunflower oil and applied as needed
reduces pain and heals herpes lesions.

CULINARY USE
Fresh leaves can be chopped into green
salad combinations or sprinkled over
fruit salad; they can also be added to
sauces, summer drinks, and desserts
as a garnish.

SAFETY INFORMATION
No issues

MENTHA SPICATA
• SPEARMINT

This erect and vigorous herb grows up to 2 ft (60 cm) in height, with tough, four-sided stems. Its pale green, wrinkled, lance-shaped leaves have serrated edges. The leaves are extremely aromatic due to the sacs within their structure that contain volatile oil. In July the plant produces small, whitish-pink flowers; if you are growing spearmint for making tea, then pinch out the flowers to encourage more leaf production. Like all mints, spearmint can be invasive once planted in a garden—it sends out suckers above ground that quickly take root. Planting it in a pot will contain it, but remember, it likes a lot of moisture and partial sun or shade.

Spearmint is a member of the vast plant family *Labiatae*, originally native to the Mediterranean. The Romans are likely to have introduced species of mint to the British Isles, along with other herbs such as lavender (see pages 150–1); these plants naturalized themselves easily. Spearmint and peppermint (see page 172–3) have a long history of use as gargles, teas, and mouthwashes. Spearmint has a sweeter, milder flavor than peppermint, and a gentler effect. Commercially distilled essential oil of spearmint makes a cooling, soothing massage remedy, especially when applied to the abdomen, easing stress-related digestive complaints.

SEE ALSO
Peppermint, fennel, cilantro, turmeric, melissa

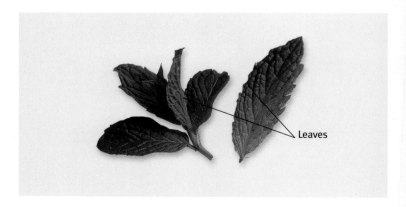

Leaves

SPEARMINT

Mentha spicata

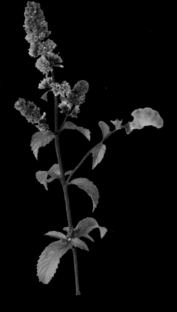

PART OF PLANT USED
Leaves

ACTIVE INGREDIENTS
Tannins, volatile oil

COMMERCIALLY AVAILABLE AS
Essential oil, tea, toothpaste

ACTIONS
Antispasmodic, digestive tonic,
carminative, febrifuge

USED TO TREAT
Indigestion, stomach cramps, gas:
tea taken after meals settles stomach
cramps and eases gas in the gut; 2 drops
of essential oil in 1 teaspoon
(5 ml) of sunflower oil massaged into the
abdomen relieves cramps.

Fever: infusion of fresh leaves, cooled,
can be used as a compress on the
forehead to ease high temperatures.
Stress-related stomach upsets: tea taken
2–3 times daily calms the mind and
eases the digestion; 2 drops of essential
oil in 1 teaspoon (5 ml) sunflower oil
massaged into the abdomen relieves
stress-related muscular tension.

CULINARY USE
Add leaves to summer punch drinks, fruit
salads or mix with cooked new potatoes.

SAFETY INFORMATION
Do not apply essential oil to sensitive,
allergy-prone skin.

MENTHA X PIPERITA
• PEPPERMINT

Peppermint is a hybrid (shown by the "*x*" in the botanical name) of two mint species: *Mentha spicata* (spearmint) and *Mentha aquatica* (water mint). It thrives in damp, heavy soil and will tolerate some shade. It is a tough, invasive plant with creeping roots, strong, four-sided, reddish stems up to 3 ft (1 m) tall and lance-shaped, slightly toothed, deep green aromatic leaves. In the summer it produces tall spikes of pinkish flowers. Once planted in a garden peppermint spreads vigorously; try controlling it by planting it in containers or in plots separated by stone boundaries (see pages 290–3). Pick leaves fresh throughout the season to use as tea or flavoring; they are best harvested in high summer for drying because the volatile oil content is strongest at that time.

It was not until the 17th century that the medicinal properties of peppermint were acknowledged in Britain, when it became hugely popular. By the 18th century it was cultivated in England as a commercial crop in Mitcham, Surrey, producing an essential oil that was considered to be the best in the world. Though this industry has declined, Germany and France have continued as commercial sources, and the United States is also a major producer of the dried herb and essential oil.

SEE ALSO
Eucalyptus, turmeric, lovage, ginger, heather

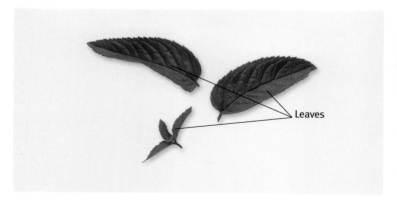

Leaves

PEPPERMINT

Mentha x piperita

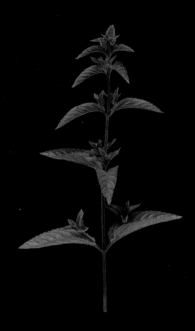

PART OF PLANT USED
Leaves

ACTIVE INGREDIENTS
Bitters, tannins, volatile oil

COMMERCIALLY AVAILABLE AS
Essential oil, toothpaste, liniment, massage balm, capsules, tea, dried herb

ACTIONS
Analgesic, antispasmodic, carminative, digestive tonic, expectorant

USED TO TREAT
Head colds, sinusitis: add 2 drops of essential oil to 2 pints (1 liter) of boiling water and inhale the steam for 10 minutes to clear blocked passages and help breathing.

Indigestion, Irritable Bowel Syndrome (IBS): capsules taken as directed ease spasms in the bowel and improve digestive rhythm.
Muscular aches and pains, rheumatism: 2 drops of essential oil added to a warm bathtub ease aches, pains and stiffness; liniment or massage balm can be massaged into affected areas afterwards for further pain relief.

CULINARY USE
Combined with sugar and vinegar, chopped peppermint makes a sauce traditionally eaten with roast lamb.

SAFETY INFORMATION
Essential oil should not be applied to sensitive or allergy-prone skin or children under the age of five.

MORUS NIGRA
• MULBERRY

The common mulberry is an attractive tree growing up to 30 ft (10 m) tall, with a dense and widely spreading canopy of branches. It bears large leaves with several lobes, and its flowers look like catkins. These turn into the fruit, which are deep red or purplish colored berries filled with juice; they resemble raspberries or loganberries, but they are larger and plumper with a tart-sweet taste. Mulberry trees can live to a great age—specimens in the grounds of stately homes in Great Britain can be as old as 500 years. Mulberry trees can be grown from seed or established from cuttings taken from older trees in early spring. They thrive in rich, well-drained soil and even do well in cities. Trees do not start producing fruit until they are at least 15 years old. In the Middle East, mulberries are dried in the sun on rooftops to preserve them over the winter.

In the 16th century the English herbalist John Gerard recommended eating raw mulberries to help sore throats and whooping cough. Mrs Grieve, in her famous *Modern Herbal* index published in 1932 gives old-fashioned recipes for mulberry wine, mulberry jam, and syrup; she makes the point that mulberry trees were grown in herb gardens to yield the luscious fruit, a concentrated source of vitamin C.

SEE ALSO
Lemon, bitter orange, grapefruit, wild strawberry, elder

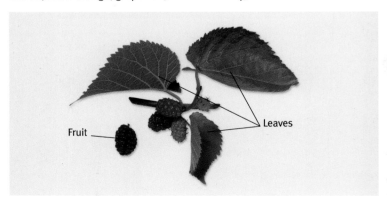

Fruit

Leaves

MULBERRY
Morus nigra

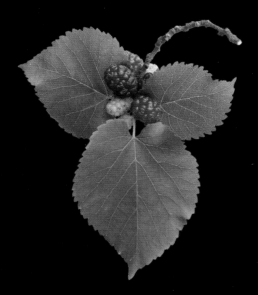

PART OF PLANT USED
Fruit

ACTIVE INGREDIENTS
Glucose, pectin, protein, vitamin C

COMMERCIALLY AVAILABLE AS
Not commercially available; mostly picked as fresh berries off trees

ACTIONS
Immune boosting, mildly laxative

USED TO TREAT
Mulberries are an example of a nutritious fruit that used to be eaten fresh and regularly preserved in jams or syrups, with tonic and immune-boosting properties. While fruit-bearing trees may not be common, the species deserves to be revisited and planted more profusely as a source of refreshing and strengthening berries and juice.

CULINARY USE
Mulberries can be eaten raw or made into jams, conserves, wine, or syrup.

SAFETY INFORMATION
No issues

MYRTUS COMMUNIS
• MYRTLE

This attractive, aromatic, evergreen shrub grows up to 10 ft (3 m) tall, with tiny, oval, glossy, dark green leaves tapering to a sharp point. Its fragrant, creamy-white flowers with a golden center bloom in July and August and small, blue-black berries form in early fall. It thrives in well-drained soil and needs plenty of nutrients; in a cooler climate it will survive frosts if set by a wall. The more it gets sun and warmth, the finer the aroma will be. Taking late summer cuttings and potting them over winter is the best way to propagate myrtle. The leaves are aromatic all year round but particularly strong smelling in July and August, so it is best to pick them at that time for drying. They retain their aroma for a long time.

Originally native to the southern Mediterranean, beautiful, sweet-smelling myrtle was considered by the ancient Greeks to be sacred to Aphrodite, the goddess of love. Myrtle flowers and leaves have long been used medicinally to treat female problems, as well as in making natural cosmetics. Even today in southern Mediterranean countries, myrtle is still included in traditional bridal bouquets, and after the wedding sprigs are planted by the new couple's home to ensure fertility and good fortune.

SEE ALSO
Bearberry/uva ursi, wild strawberry, eucalyptus, tea tree, bitter orange

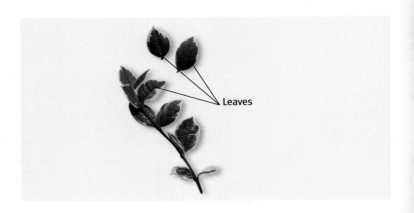

Leaves

MYRTLE
Myrtus communis

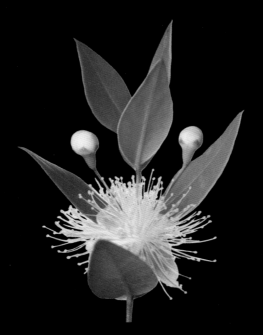

PART OF PLANT USED
Leaves

ACTIVE INGREDIENTS
Volatile oil

COMMERCIALLY AVAILABLE AS
Essential oil, massage balm

ACTIONS
Antiseptic, expectorant, immune stimulant

USED TO TREAT
Urinary tract infections: 2 drops of essential oil added to a warm bathtub soothes irritation and fights urinary infections.
Coughs and colds: add 2 drops of essential oil to 1 pint (500 ml) of boiling water and inhale the steam for 10 minutes to ease breathing; 2 drops of essential oil in 1 teaspoon (5 ml) of sunflower oil massaged into the chest morning and night also helps breathing and improves sleep.
Oily, combination, or mature skin: 2 drops of essential oil in 1 teaspoon (5 ml) of aloe vera gel applied night and morning tones the pores and balances oil production in the upper skin layers.

CULINARY USE
In Middle Eastern countries dried myrtle berries are used to flavor strong-tasting meats such as game.

SAFETY INFORMATION
No issues

OCIMUM BASILICUM
• BASIL

A wonderfully aromatic annual herb, basil grows approximately 8–24 in (20–60 cm) tall. Garden centers supply several well-known varieties: *Ocimum basilicum var. "Genovese"* is compact and highly aromatic; *var. "Purple Ruffles"* has dark leaves that smell of cloves; *var. "Minimum"* is very small and good for growing on window ledges; and the vigorous *var. "Crispum"* has curly leaves. The classic species can be grown from seed and planted in pots in moist, loamy soil in full sun; in more northern climates it does well on a window ledge or in a conservatory. It produces highly aromatic stems and leaves. In summer spikes of tiny white flowers appear, so to maximize leaf production, pinch out flowering stalks—this gives a steady supply of delicious leaves all through the season.

The fragrance of basil has been enjoyed for centuries. The 17th-century English herbalist John Parkinson regarded it as one of the best herbs to make fragrant toilet waters, and said that the aroma alone was fit to scent the house of a king. In India a variety of basil called "*Ocimum sanctum*" (holy basil) is given the Sanksrit name "*tulsi*," and is frequently planted in gardens to ward off misfortune, being considered sacred to the god Vishnu.

SEE ALSO
Eucalyptus, myrtle, senna, dill, tea tree

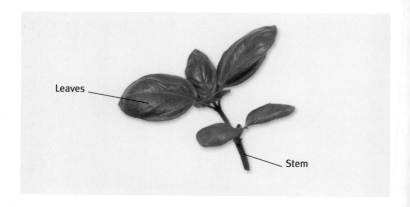

Leaves

Stem

BASIL

Ocimum basilicum

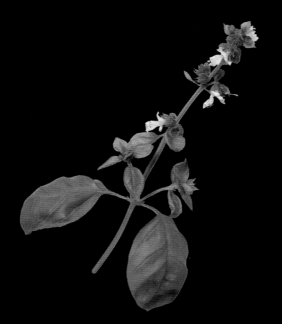

PART OF PLANT USED
Leaves

ACTIVE INGREDIENTS
Glycosides, saponins, tannins, volatile oil

COMMERCIALLY AVAILABLE AS
Dried and fresh herb, essential oil, tincture

ACTIONS
Antiseptic, antispasmodic, emmenagogue, expectorant

USED TO TREAT
Blocked sinuses, head colds: add 2 drops of essential oil to 17 fl oz (500 ml) of boiling water and inhale the steam for 10 minutes to ease breathing.
Chesty coughs: an infusion of fresh leaves with a teaspoon of honey, drunk 2–3 times daily, eases coughs.
Indigestion, constipation: an infusion of fresh leaves taken after meals settles the digestion and improves bowel rhythm.
Insect bites or stings: rub fresh leaves onto bites and stings to soothe them.

CULINARY USE
Add fresh leaves to green or tomato salads; it is a classic ingredient in pesto sauce and often used in Italian cooking.

SAFETY INFORMATION
Basil essential oil should be avoided in pregnancy as it can encourage menstruation. Eating leaves as a flavoring, however, is safe.

OENOTHERA BIENNIS
• EVENING PRIMROSE

This tall plant grows up to 5 ft (1.5 m) in height. It is biennial, which means it completes its growing cycle in two years, flowering in the second year. Evening primrose has a thick, yellow taproot and a rosette of leaves at the base from which the flower stalks rise. It has narrow, dark green leaves, and scented yellow flowers forming in clusters, opening at night to attract pollinators. Downy pods form after the flowers fall, and contain the seeds. Evening primrose tolerates most soils, and likes a warm, sunny position. Once established, it will self-seed freely. Evening primrose is now farmed commercially for the extraction of the fatty oil from the seeds that is sold as a nutritional supplement.

The plant was originally native to North America. It was imported to Italy in the 17th century and it then naturalized itself throughout Europe. In the late 20th century, clinical research identified significant amounts of gamma-linolenic acid (GLA) in the seeds. This compound has a significant effect on levels of prostoglandins (hormone-like substances) and therefore influences hormone balance. Research in Europe and the United States has since highlighted many benefits of evening primrose oil, including skin enhancing properties and healing effects on eczema.

SEE ALSO
Agnus castus, black cohosh, sage, clary sage, borage

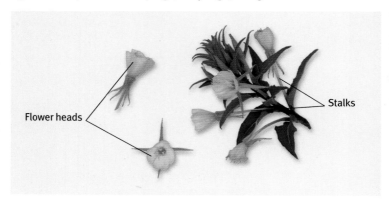

Flower heads

Stalks

EVENING PRIMROSE

Oenothera biennis

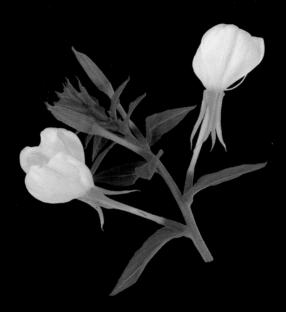

PART OF PLANT USED
Seeds

ACTIVE INGREDIENTS
GLA (gamma-linoleic acid) and other
fatty acids

COMMERCIALLY AVAILABLE AS
Capsules, liquid oil, face cream,
skin cream

ACTIONS
Hormone balancing, skin-rejuvenating,
vulnerary

USED TO TREAT
PMS, period pain, irregular periods:
capsules taken as directed, for at least
three months, reduce period pain and
ease bloating and other pre-menstrual
discomfort, as well as regulating cycles.
*Menopausal transition and
symptoms (hot flashes):* long-term
supplementation with capsules
as directed reduces symptoms by
regulating hormone balance.
Eczema, dry, damaged, or mature skin:
pierce a capsule with a needle, squeeze
out the oil and apply directly onto an
affected area, twice daily, to speed
healing and improve skin texture.

CULINARY USE
None

SAFETY INFORMATION
Although a study in the early 1980s
suggested it should be avoided by
epileptics, recent research has shown
that this can be disregarded.

OLEA EUROPEA
• OLIVE

A tough, evergreen tree growing up to 40 ft (12 m) in height, the olive tree has a pale gray bark, and long, smooth, leathery green leaves. Its cream-colored flowers are followed by the fruit—olives—which ripen to dark purple. Native to the Mediterranean and the Middle East, olive trees thrive in well-drained soil and intense heat. If planted in cooler climates, they will resist frost but they will not produce fruit. In countries that commercially produce olives the fruit is picked green for pressing because it is less acid, which improves the quality of the olive oil. First pressed "extra virgin" olive oil has the finest flavor and highest vitamin and mineral content.

Olive trees have been cultivated for thousands of years. The name "olive" comes from the Latin "*oleum*" meaning oil. A vital commodity, olive oil has been used continuously in cooking and cosmetics right up to the present day. In recent years, scientific analysis of olive leaves has highlighted several important compounds with antiseptic, antimicrobial, and antiviral properties, and olive leaf extract is now available as an effective immune-supportive supplement.

SEE ALSO

Hawthorn, Devil's claw, turmeric, borage, echinacea

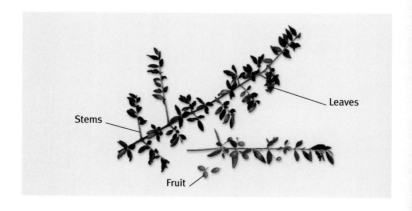

Leaves

Stems

Fruit

OLIVE

Olea europea

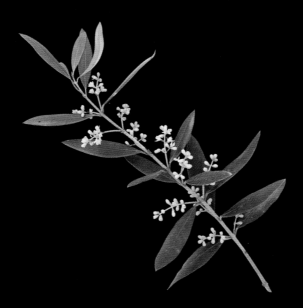

PARTS OF PLANT USED
Fruit, leaves

ACTIVE INGREDIENTS
Fruit—vitamin E, oleic acid
Leaves—tannins, oleuropein

COMMERCIALLY AVAILABLE AS
Oil, leaf extract in capsules and
liquid form; oil used in soaps,
shampoos, creams

ACTIONS
Oil—cholesterol-lowering, skin
rejuvenating; leaf extract—antiseptic,
antimicrobial, antiviral

USED TO TREAT
*High blood pressure due to high
cholesterol:* consuming 1 fl oz (30 g) of
extra virgin olive oil in the diet daily can
lower blood cholesterol.
*Constipation, Irritable Bowel Syndrome
(IBS):* regular dietary use regulates the
colon and soothes the bowel lining.
Dry, dehydrated skin: apply extra-virgin
olive oil regularly to improve skin
suppleness and elasticity.
Influenza, glandular fever, viruses; olive-
leaf extract taken as directed increases
immune-system responses to viral
infections, so symptoms clear quickly.

CULINARY USE
It is a vital ingredient in salad dressings,
sauces, and Mediterranean cooking.

SAFETY INFORMATION
People with high blood pressure should
discuss the use of olive oil with a doctor.

ORIGANUM MARJORANA
• MARJORAM

This low-growing, perennial herb produces a mat of foliage made up of small, broad, lance-shaped, aromatic, green leaves. It produces spikes of tiny pink flowers in late summer. It requires moist, well-drained soil in full sun. It can be grown from seed in the spring but will not resist frost, so cover and protect plants the following fall, or plant marjoram in pots to bring indoors over winter. If you grow marjoram as a culinary herb, pinch out flower stalks to maximize leaf production for culinary use. Leaves can be harvested throughout the growing season and added to dishes or brewed as a tea.

The botanical name "*Origanum*" comes from a Greek phrase "*oros ganos*," meaning "joy of the mountain"—this shows the Mediterranean origin of the plant. Marjoram is closely related to oregano (see pages 186–7), also used in Greek and Italian cooking, but can easily be distinguished because the former is low growing and has darker green leaves. Marjoram has been grown as a medicinal and culinary herb since ancient Egyptian times and was known to the Greeks and Romans; the latter are most likely to have introduced it to Britain.

SEE ALSO
Black cohosh, rosemary, heather, lavender, melissa

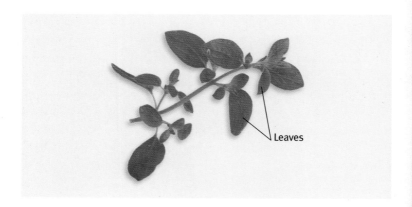

Leaves

MARJORAM

Origanum marjorana

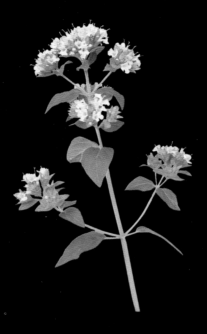

PART OF PLANT USED
Leaves

ACTIVE INGREDIENTS
Bitters, carotenes, tannins, vitamin C,
volatile oil

COMMERCIALLY AVAILABLE AS
Dried and fresh herb, essential oil

ACTIONS
Antispasmodic, digestive tonic, sedative

USED TO TREAT
Menstrual pain: 2 drops of essential oil
added to 1 teaspoon (5 ml) of sunflower
oil, massaged into the abdomen 2–3
times daily, eases cramps; an infusion of
fresh leaves can also be drunk 2–3 times
daily to improve relaxation and sleep.

Muscular aches and pains, rheumatism:
2 drops of essential oil added to a warm
bathtub relieves pain and stiffness.
Insomnia, anxiety: an infusion of fresh
leaves eases anxiety and increases
relaxation; 2 drops of essential oil added
to a warm bathtub is relaxing.
Stress-related indigestion: 2 drops of
essential oil added to 1 teaspoon
(5 ml) of sunflower oil massaged into the
abdomen twice daily soothes anxiety.

CULINARY USE
Marjoram is used in Mediterranean and
Middle Eastern cuisine to flavor sauces,
and meat and fish dishes.

SAFETY INFORMATION
No issues

ORIGANUM VULGARE
• OREGANO

This bushy, perennial herb grows up to 2 ft (60 cm) tall with highly aromatic, small, lance-shaped leaves. It produces stalks of tiny, pinkish-purple flowers in late summer and is very attractive to bees, butterflies, and other beneficial insects. Native to the southern Mediterranean, it is a tough survivor and grows well in rocky coastal locations, thriving in sandy, well-drained soil and hot sunshine. It is best propagated from cuttings taken in the spring, matured in pots, and then planted out the following year. For culinary or medicinal use, pick fresh leaves throughout the season or gather the flowering tops in August or September to dry for later use.

In ancient Greece oregano was considered an effective remedy against poisoning and convulsions and as a poultice for deep wounds. The Romans believed oregano brought joy and good fortune to married couples, so it was made into bridal wreaths at weddings. Its powerful aroma made it popular in medieval times as a "strewing herb" mixed into the straw commonly used as a floor covering.

SEE ALSO
Yellow gentian, valerian, lavender, juniper, goldenseal

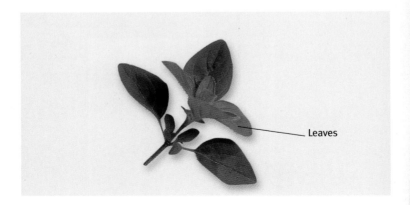

Leaves

OREGANO

Origanum vulgare

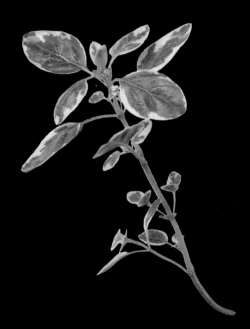

PART OF PLANT USED
Leaves

ACTIVE INGREDIENTS
Bitters, tannins, volatile oil

COMMERCIALLY AVAILABLE AS
Essential oil, fresh or dried herb

ACTIONS
Antispasmodic, astringent, expectorant, sedative

USED TO TREAT
Indigestion of rich foods, liver and gall-bladder problems: an infusion of fresh or dried leaves taken after meals stimulates liver and gallbladder function.
Insomnia: an infusion of fresh or dried leaves, taken in the evening with a spoonful of honey, calms anxiety and improves relaxation.
Muscular aches and pains, rheumatism: 2 drops of essential oil added to 1 teaspoon (5 ml) of sunflower oil massaged into affected areas 2–3 times daily, warms and eases muscles.
Cuts and wounds: a strong infusion of fresh leaves, still warm, makes a useful compress solution to draw dirt out of fresh cuts or wounds.

CULINARY USE
Fresh oregano is traditionally added to a Greek salad, as well as to many Italian recipes, including pizza.

SAFETY INFORMATION
Do not use essential oil in pregnancy; culinary use of the herb, however, is safe.

PANAX GINSENG
• GINSENG

One of the most popular herbal tonics in the world, ginseng is known as "*ren shen*" in Chinese, which means "man root" — its thick, yellowish roots sometimes resemble human figures. Above ground the plant can grow up to 2 ft (60 cm) tall with finely divided leaves, and produces a single umbel of yellow flowers and bright red berries. Many grades and types of ginseng exist. Manchurian or wild ginseng from China is considered the best quality, though very expensive. Cultivated ginseng comes in two types, red or white, mostly from Korea. The red type is cured by steaming, which gives it the color and also makes it more stimulating than the white. American ginseng (*Panax quinquefolium*) has a milder effect and less potent ingredients.

Traditional Chinese medicine regards ginseng as an important tonic for older people, and often blends it with other herbs to balance its potent effects. It is particularly popular in China as a seasonal remedy, taken in the fall to help the transition into winter. In the west ginseng has gained huge popularity as an "adaptogenic" herb, because of its steroid-like compounds. This means it can be either a sedative or a stimulant, taken to energize the body or help combat stress. However if stress is a major problem, simply taking ginseng will not solve it — considering lifestyle changes is important too.

SEE ALSO
Ginger, cardamom, black pepper, garlic, bitter orange

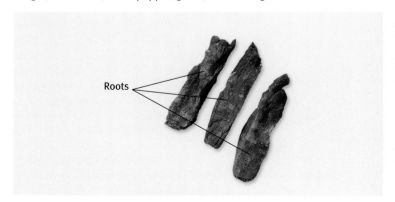

Roots

GINSENG
Panax ginseng

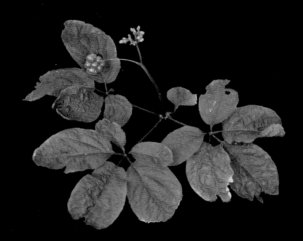

189

PART OF PLANT USED
Roots

ACTIVE INGREDIENTS
Hormone-like saponins, minerals, sterols, starch, sugar, vitamins, volatile oil

COMMERCIALLY AVAILABLE AS
Capsules, tablets, tea

ACTIONS
Adaptogenic, tonic

USED TO TREAT
Convalescence after illness: tablets or capsules taken as directed for about a month after a period of illness help to rebuild physical strength and vitality.
Low energy, physical and mental stress, low libido: tablets or capsules taken as directed for 1–2 months can increase energy levels; however, consider lifestyle changes as well to lower stress.

CULINARY USE
None

SAFETY INFORMATION
Avoid in pregnancy because of its potent stimulating and hormonal effects. Avoid taking caffeine-rich drinks if using ginseng as these will over-stress the nervous system. Avoid ginseng during episodes of bronchitis as its stimulating effect can worsen symptoms.

PASSIFLORA INCARNATA
• PASSION FLOWER

This hardy perennial is a climbing plant, best trained up a trellis or a fence, where it can reach up to 26 ft (8 m) if left to grow freely. It has deeply lobed, dark leaves and clings to support with strong tendrils. Its flowers are made up of pale pink or purple "fingers," and its central stamens form a stunning geometric green shape. Native to the United States, this species of passion flower is now cultivated commercially in Virginia, Kentucky, Florida, Texas, and Arizona. It requires well-drained, sandy soil and a very sunny position, sheltered from cold winds in cooler climates. It can be propagated using cuttings in the late summer, and it is also easily sourced from garden suppliers. The flowers are the active medicinal part; they are dried and used in many commercial herbal-tablet or tea blends to help insomnia.

The flower acquired its common and botanical names because of the cross in the center of its flower, seen as symbolic of the crucifixion that is referred to as the Passion of Christ. The internal structures of the flower also resemble nails. Different species of passiflora are found both in North and South America; *Passiflora incarnata* was used by Native American people as a nerve tonic.

SEE ALSO
Melissa, lavender, valerian, hops, Roman camomile

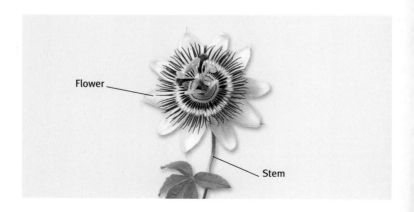

Flower

Stem

PASSION FLOWER

Passiflora incarnata

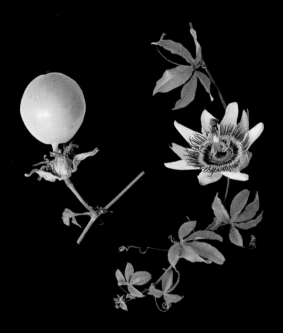

PART OF PLANT USED
Flowers

ACTIVE INGREDIENTS
Alkaloids, flavonoids, gum,
sterols, sugar

COMMERCIALLY AVAILABLE AS
Tea, capsules, tablets

ACTIONS
Hypotensive, nerve tonic, sedative

USED TO TREAT
Insomnia: tablets or capsules taken as
directed, or tea taken in the late evening,
all help to relax the mind and improve
sleep quality.
Mental stress, anxiety, nervous tension:
tablets or capsules taken as directed

have a sedative effect on the mind,
easing stress and worry.
High blood pressure: tablets or capsules
taken as directed can help reduce high
blood pressure.

CULINARY USE
None

SAFETY INFORMATION
If you are on prescribed medication
such as tranquilizers, or suffer from high
blood pressure, please consult a doctor
or a qualified medical herbalist before
using passion flower.

PETROSELINUM CRISPUM
• PARSLEY

A biennial herb growing from a stout root, parsley grows up to 2 ft (60 cm) tall, producing triangular, three-lobed leaves with very curled ends, giving it a "ruffled" appearance. Umbels of yellow flowers bloom in the second year after planting, followed by oval seed pods containing sickle-shaped seeds. Seed is best sown in the late spring. Originally native to the Mediterranean, parsley is now widely cultivated in many varieties. It needs rich, moist, well-drained soil in a sunny position; as a kitchen herb, it grows easily in pots, yielding a steady supply of fresh leaves.

The Greek physician Dioscorides gave this plant the name "*Petroselinum*" in the 1st century CE, derived from the Greek "*petra*" (rock) and "*selinon*" (celery). Fresh leaves are popular in cooking to this day—their strong taste can even neutralize garlic. The seeds are used in herbal medicine; however, they are very diuretic and remedies made with them should only be used under professional guidance. They are often combined with other digestive herbs.

SEE ALSO
Yellow gentian, licorice, peppermint, horsetail fern, Devil's claw

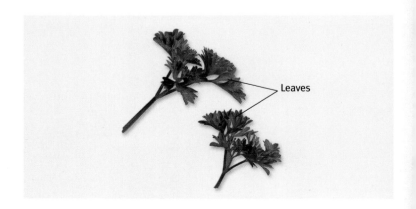

Leaves

PARSLEY

Petroselinum crispum

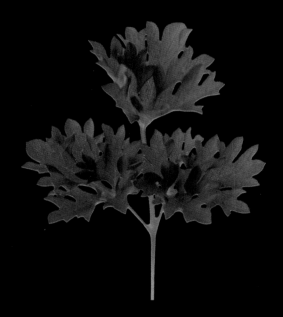

PART OF PLANT USED
Leaves, seeds

ACTIVE INGREDIENTS
Leaves — iron, vitamin C; seeds — volatile oil

COMMERCIALLY AVAILABLE AS
Fresh or dried herb, tablets, capsules

ACTIONS
Antispasmodic, carminative, digestive tonic, diuretic, emmenagogue

USED TO TREAT
Indigestion of rich foods: leaves eaten as garnish or brewed as an infusion taken after a meal help to settle the stomach.
Anemia: leaves eaten freely in the diet are rich in iron, providing a natural tonic.

Fluid retention, gout, urinary-tract infections: seeds taken in capsules or tablets have a strong diuretic effect, helping to detoxify the system.
Rheumatism: seeds taken in tablets or capsules taken as directed help with detoxification and internal cleansing.

CULINARY USE
Leaves make a visually attractive and nutritious garnish in salads, on egg or cheese dishes, and in soups and sauces.

SAFETY INFORMATION
Parsley-seed remedies should not be used in pregnancy, because they can stimulate menstruation; if you are taking diuretic or anti-rheumatic medication, please consult a doctor or medical herbalist before using parsley seed.

PINUS SYLVESTRIS
• PINE

This species—also known as Scots or Norway pine—is one of a vast family of trees, native to and commercially cultivated in many countries across Europe, Scandinavia, North America, and Canada. *Pinus sylvestris* is grown for timber production and its thin leaves—called needles—yield a pungent and fresh-smelling essential oil by distillation. The tree has a vertical trunk and grows up to 100 ft (30 m) tall, with a crown of needle foliage, and produces cones containing small seeds. Like all pine species, the tree is very hardy and grows to full height relatively quickly, tolerating cold winters and harsh weather.

In the past, in northern European countries such as Germany and Switzerland, pine resin that oozed out of the bark was used as an expectorant—dissolved in hot water, either in the bathtub or inhaled to help respiratory problems. Today pine essential oil is very commonly used as a natural fragrance in the commercial production of toiletries, shampoos, and cleaning products; it is also a common ingredient in pharmaceutical preparations such as liniments or ointments for aches and pains, or lozenges and medicines for coughs.

SEE ALSO
Rosemary, black pepper, ginger, cayenne, eucalyptus

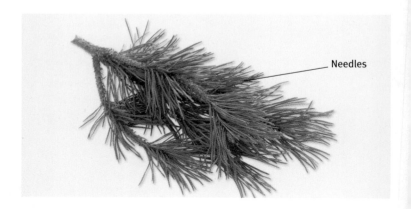

Needles

PINE

Pinus sylvestris

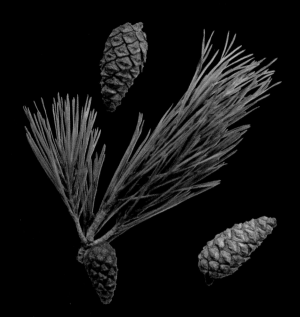

PART OF PLANT USED
Needles (leaves)

ACTIVE INGREDIENTS
Volatile oil

COMMERCIALLY AVAILABLE AS
Liniment, ointment, massage balm, cough medicine, lozenges, essential oil, shampoos, bath products

ACTIONS
Analgesic, expectorant, local circulation stimulant

USED TO TREAT
Muscular aches and pains, rheumatism: add 2 drops of essential oil to a bathtub or to 1 teaspoon (5 ml) of sunflower oil, then massage into affected areas.

Poor circulation: 2 drops of essential oil in 1 teaspoon (5 ml) of sunflower oil massaged into affected areas as needed will improve circulation and ease inner chills; liniment or massage balm applied as directed helps in the same way.
Colds and coughs: add 2 drops of essential oil to 17 fl oz (500 ml) of boiling water and inhale the steam vapor for 10 minutes to clear the chest and help breathing; lozenges or cough medicine taken as directed also ease the chest.

CULINARY USE
None

SAFETY INFORMATION
Do not use essential oil on sensitive or skin, or on children under the age of five.

PIPER METHYSTICUM
• KAVA KAVA

This plant is native to Polynesia and the islands of the South Seas; it is a member of the same family as black pepper (see pages 198–9). Kava kava is a shrub growing up to 6ft (2 m) in height, with heavily veined leaves and small spikes of flowers produced where the leaf stalks meet the main stem. The thick root, or rhizome, is the active medicinal part—in native tradition, sections of the root are dug up and chewed, and then mixed with water or coconut juice to make a special drink, which gives a feeling of well-being and euphoria.

Interest in kava kava was raised in the 1980s, when people began taking it as a supplement to improve mood. However, between 2003 and 2005, food and drug agencies in the United States, Great Britain, Europe, and Australia decided to restrict its sale to the general public—in Great Britain, it is completely banned from retail outlets. This is because concerns were raised about instances of associated liver damage in a small number of individuals worldwide. Though the evidence against kava kava is by no means conclusive, and it is still widely available online via Internet-based herbal suppliers, it is best to consult a qualified herbalist if you are interested in taking it.

SEE ALSO

Bearberry/uva ursi, fennel, saw palmetto, yarrow, angelica

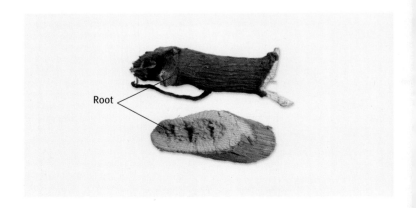

Root

KAVA KAVA

Piper methysticum

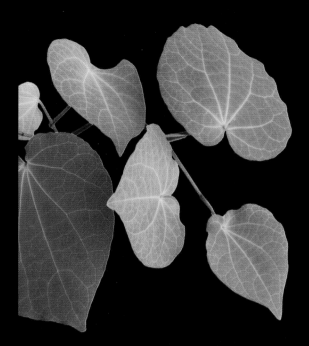

PART OF PLANT USED
Roots

ACTIVE INGREDIENTS
Alkaloids, oleo-resin (including kavalactones), mucilage, starch

COMMERCIALLY AVAILABLE AS
Not available through retail outlets in Great Britain; limited retail availability as capsules or teas in Australia; available online in the United States

ACTIONS
Anti-inflammatory, diuretic

USED TO TREAT
Bladder, urinary and prostate problems: kava kava should only be used to help these issues under the guidance of a professional medical herbalist.
Rheumatism, gout: capsules or external application of kava kava extract should only be undertaken with professional guidance, as above.

CULINARY USE
None

SAFETY INFORMATION
Kava kava should not be taken in pregnancy because of its strong effects on the nervous system. Also anyone with medically diagnosed urinary or rheumatic problems should consult a doctor or medical herbalist before using it.

PIPER NIGRUM
• BLACK PEPPER

This vigorous plant is a vine that can grow up to 24 ft (8 m) in height and spread. It has a very tough, woody stem and produces many heart-shaped, shiny, dark green leaves. Native to India, Malaysia, and Indonesia, pepper plants need deep, rich, well-fertilized soil, full sun and a humid, tropical atmosphere. They will grow in heated greenhouses or conservatories in cooler climates, but will not flower—and they need regular spraying with water to keep the leaves moist. In the intense heat of their native environment, small drooping clusters of tiny, white flowers become the peppercorns, which are red as they mature; left in the sun they turn black. White pepper is produced from the ripe dried berries with the black husk removed. Black peppercorns contain the maximum amount of volatile oil giving them the most pungent flavor.

In ancient times, spices such as pepper were very rare, and considered as valuable as gold. Pepper arrived in western Europe during the Middle Ages thanks to the opening of trade routes to India and later Malaysia.

SEE ALSO

Cardamom, turmeric, lemon, dill, rosemary, bay laurel

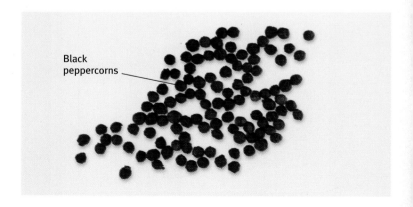

Black peppercorns

BLACK PEPPER

Piper nigrum

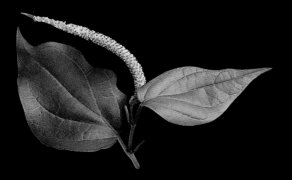

PART OF PLANT USED
Fruit (peppercorns)

ACTIVE INGREDIENTS
Volatile oil

COMMERCIALLY AVAILABLE AS
Essential oil, dried peppercorns, massage balm

ACTIONS
Analgesic, antiviral, digestive tonic, local circulation stimulant

USED TO TREAT
Influenza, viral infections: 2 drops of essential oil in a bathtub twice daily soothes and strengthens the body.
Colds, coughs: add 2 drops of essential oil to 1 teaspoon (5 ml) of sunflower oil to massage the chest area 2–3 times daily; this helps breathing.
Indigestion, constipation: add 2 drops of essential oil to 1 teaspoon (5 ml) of sunflower oil and massage the abdomen in a clockwise, circular direction, to help indigestion and loosen the bowel.
Muscular aches and pains, arthritis, rheumatism, stiff joints: 2 drops of essential oil in 1 teaspoon (5 ml) of sunflower oil massaged into affected areas twice daily eases sore muscles.

CULINARY USE
Freshly ground black pepper is a key spice in most savory dishes.

SAFETY INFORMATION
Do not use essential oil on sensitive skin, or on children under the age of five.

PRIMULA VERA
• COWSLIP

This herb is an example of a plant that used to be found growing wild all over Britain and northern Europe (the United States has various native species of *Primula*, some with similar uses). However, with the increased use of commercial pesticides in European farming, cowslip is becoming much rarer, and some countries have designated it a protected species. Seeds can be obtained from horticultural suppliers—by growing it yourself, you are helping the species to survive. Cowslip is a low-growing plant up to 9 in (24 cm) tall, with a short, stout root. It needs rich, moist soil. It produces long, wrinkled, hairy, oval leaves, with erect, flowering stems in the center; rosettes of small, deep yellow flowers form in umbel-shaped clusters, and have a sweet scent. The flowers are mostly used medicinally and need to be harvested just as they are opening. The root is sometimes dug up and dried to make a remedy for coughs.

Hundreds of years ago cowslip flowers were used to brew a potent country wine, as they contain mild amounts of a narcotic with an uplifting effect on the mind. The flowers were also used to make a tea to help headaches and restlessness, or made into face creams and washes for cosmetic use. Cowslip was so widespread that it was a true example of a "people's remedy."

SEE ALSO
Goldenseal, white horehound, myrrh, lavender, melissa

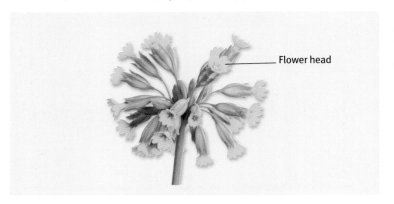

Flower head

COWSLIP
Primula vera

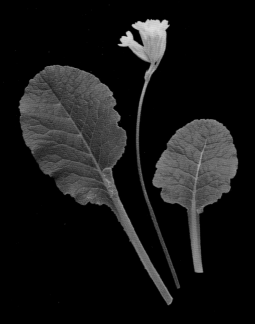

PARTS OF PLANT USED:
Flowers, roots

ACTIVE INGREDIENTS
Flowers — flavonoids, saponins, volatile oil; root — glycosides, saponins

COMMERCIALLY AVAILABLE AS
Dried flowers, teas, cough medicine, liquid herbal tonic, lozenges

ACTIONS
Diuretic, expectorant, sedative

USED TO TREAT
Coughs, chest congestion: cough medicine or lozenges taken as directed soothe the respiratory tract as well as helping to expel catarrh.
Headaches, anxiety, nervous tension: an infusion of fresh or dried flowers taken 2–3 times daily calms the nervous system.
Insomnia: an infusion of fresh or dried flowers taken before bed helps to relax the mind.
Inflamed joints, arthritis: in mainland Europe, cowslip root is a very popular liquid herb tonic taken to ease inflammation of the joints.

CULINARY USE
Flowers can be candied as cake decorations.

SAFETY INFORMATION
No issues

PULMONARIA OFFICINALIS
• LUNGWORT

A member of the same plant family as borage (see pages 62–3) this perennial herb grows up to 1 ft (30 cm) in height. It produces a slightly hairy stem with angled, alternate leaves, which are long and lance-shaped, covered with tiny hairs and speckled with whitish dots. The flowers are small, blue and pink, bell-like blooms in clusters. Lungwort grows wild in many parts of Europe, in woodland, hedgerows, and waste ground. It is not native to Britain but it has established itself there. It needs partial shade and a moist soil, and it can easily be sown from seed. The leaves and flowers are the medicinal part of the plant, collected as the flowers come into bloom.

Both the botanical and common names of the plant—"*Pulmonaria*" and "lungwort"—refer directly to the lungs. In ancient times, a medical theory known as the "doctrine of signatures" held that plants that resembled parts of the body would be useful treatments for their ailments—because the fleshy appearance of lungwort resembled lung tissue, it was named for the lungs and used to treat respiratory problems. Lungwort contains a large amount of mucilage, a thick, gel-like substance with a soothing and anti-inflammatory effect on the inner lining of the respiratory tract. It is still used today as an important ingredient in commercial herbal cough mixtures.

SEE ALSO
White horehound, daisy, manuka, echinacea, witch hazel

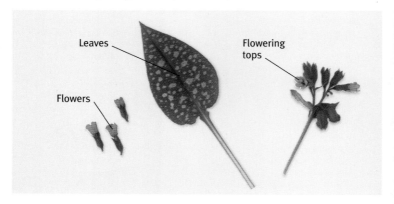

Leaves

Flowering tops

Flowers

LUNGWORT

Pulmonaria officinalis

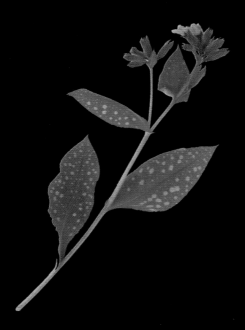

PARTS OF PLANT USED
Leaves and flowers

ACTIVE INGREDIENTS
Alkaloids, mineral salts, mucilage, saponins, tannins

COMMERCIALLY AVAILABLE AS
Cough medicine

ACTIONS
Anti-inflammatory, astringent, emollient, expectorant

USED TO TREAT
Tickly coughs: cough medicine taken as directed soothes the lining of the respiratory tract, easing irritation.
Bronchitis, chest congestion or inflammation: cough medicine taken as directed eases deep, chesty coughs and loosens catarrh.
Wounds, cuts, damaged skin: an infusion of fresh leaves, cooled, makes an astringent and anti-inflammatory skin wash to cleanse damaged skin and slow bleeding.

CULINARY USE
None

SAFETY INFORMATION
The particular alkaloid content of lungwort has led to its restriction in some countries because of anxieties over possible side effects on the liver if taken internally—if in doubt check with a professional herbal practitioner.

QUERCUS ROBUR
• OAK

A large deciduous tree growing up to 150 ft (50 m) tall, oak trees produce a thick trunk and massive branches, to a full potential width of 100 ft (30 m). They can live for hundreds of years and some specimens have achieved a trunk circumference of up to 90 ft (30 m). They produce leathery and dark green leaves, typically with multi-lobed edges. Male flowers (catkins) and female flowers appear together, leading to the formation of the acorn, the fruit of the oak. Oak bark is the medicinal part of the tree—in the past it has also been used as a dye and to tan leather.

The oak tree is a significant ancient symbol, bound up with the history of the British Isles for more than 1,000 years. The druids, an ancient priesthood, were said to have held their gatherings in groves of oak trees. Oak timber is among the hardest woods in the world, extensively used in the past for shipbuilding and house frames. Today, oak bark is used in herbal medicine to treat diarrhea and various skin problems. Oak is also part of the Bach flower remedy system, used to combat stress.

SEE ALSO
Cayenne, black pepper, horse chestnut, witch hazel, St. John's wort

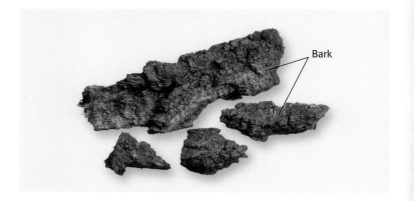

Bark

OAK

Quercus robur

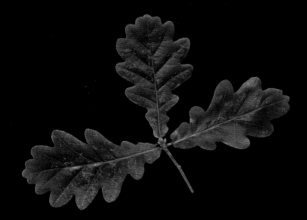

PART OF PLANT USED
Bark

ACTIVE INGREDIENTS
Tannins

COMMERCIALLY AVAILABLE AS
Dried bark, hemorrhoid ointment,
flower remedy

ACTIONS
Antiseptic, astringent

USED TO TREAT
Cold limbs, chilblains: a decoction (see
page 297) of the dried bark boiled in
water and cooled can be applied as a
compress or added to a bathtub to help
the circulation.
Hemorrhoids: ointment applied as

directed is a natural astringent, helping
to shrink enlarged veins in the rectum.
Diarrhea: 3 fl oz (100 ml) of decoction
drunk 2–3 times daily can help to ease
diarrhea spasms.
Mental and physical overload: oak
flower remedy taken 2–3 times daily
eases the burden of physical and
mental effort in people who tend to
take on too much.

CULINARY USE
None

SAFETY INFORMATION
No issues; the bark is most likely to
be freely available from a professional
herbal practitioner.

RIBES NIGRUM
• BLACKCURRANT

This fragrant, deciduous shrub is a good choice as a fruit-bearing and medicinally helpful garden plant. It grows up to 4 ft (1.2 m) tall with long, erect, thin twigs and alternate three- or five-lobed, dark green leaves, coarsely toothed at the edges. The flowers are greenish white and are produced in the axils where the leaf stems join the main stem. These change into the familiar blue-black berry known as the blackcurrant. All parts of the plant have a very pleasant, sharp and sweet aroma. Blackcurrant bushes can make a useful and attractive hedge in a garden; they thrive in well-drained, nutrient-rich soil and need plenty of moisture.

The blackcurrant was originally native to Asia and northern and central Europe; it has now spread throughout Europe, Great Britain, and the United States through cultivation. The medicinal use of blackcurrant dates back to the 16th century, when the leaves were infused as a tonic for rheumatism. Today, most commercial, medicinal and cosmetic interest is in the fatty oil from the seeds, which is rich in GLA (gamma-linoleic acid), also found in evening primrose (see pages 180–1) and borage seed (see pages 62–3).

SEE ALSO
Lemon, myrtle, heather, evening primrose, borage

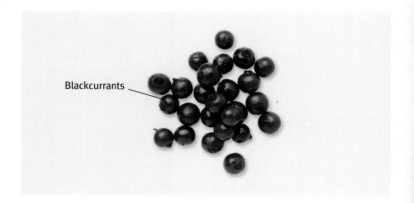

Blackcurrants

BLACKCURRANT

Ribes nigrum

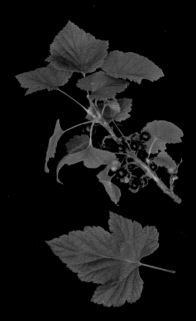

PARTS OF PLANT USED
Fruit, leaves, seeds

ACTIVE INGREDIENTS
Fruit—vitamin C; leaves—organic acids, sugar, tannins, volatile oil; seeds—gamma-linoleic acid (GLA)

COMMERCIALLY AVAILABLE AS
Juice or jam from fruit; tea in herbal mixtures; seed oil capsules

ACTIONS
Fruit—immune tonic; leaves—diuretic, cleansing; seeds—skin rejuvenating, hormone balancing

USED TO TREAT
Low immunity, colds, coughs: fresh berries or juice taken twice daily strengthen the immune system.
Rheumatism: infusion of blackcurrant leaves taken 2–3 times daily has an internally cleansing effect.
Urinary-tract infections: infusion of leaves taken 2–3 times daily helps the kidneys detoxify the body.
Dry or mature skin: capsules taken as directed help to improve skin texture; oil can be directly applied to the skin.
PMS/menopausal problems: seed-oil capsules taken as directed for a minimum three-month period help to rebalance hormones and energy levels.

CULINARY USE
Jams, jellies, conserves, and juices

SAFETY INFORMATION
No issues

ROSA CANINA
• ROSE HIP

This originally wild-growing shrub is also known as the dog rose (the meaning of the botanical name). It grows wild throughout Europe and Great Britain, in hedgerows, scrubland, and woods. It does well in rich soils but can tolerate poorer conditions, though it does need plenty of moisture. It grows up to 6 ft (2 m) tall with strong, downward-curving branches covered in stout prickles. The leafing stalks end in five or seven small leaflets with serrated edges. The flowers, which bloom in June and July, have either white or pale pink petals, and a sweet scent. In the early fall, the fruit forms—these are bright red "rose hips."

For hundreds of years, wild rose hips have provided a valuable source of vitamin C to rural people, who picked them in the fall to make into tea or syrup to be used during the winter to help coughs and colds in adults and children. In recent years, research in Germany has shown that taking rose hip as a supplement is a natural anti-inflammatory and antioxidant remedy for osteoarthritis and rheumatoid arthritis, reducing the need for conventional pain relief.

SEE ALSO
Garlic, echinacea, bearberry/uva ursi, carrot seed, Devil's claw

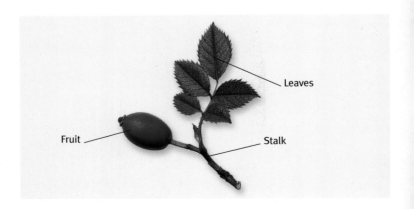

Leaves

Fruit

Stalk

ROSE HIP

Rosa canina

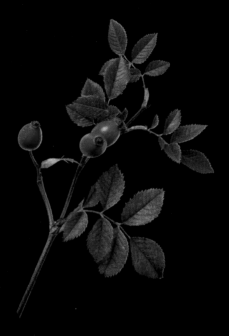

PART OF PLANT USED
Fruit ("hips")

ACTIVE INGREDIENTS
Fatty oil, glycosides, tannins, vitamin C, volatile oil

COMMERCIALLY AVAILABLE AS
Tablets, capsules, teas

ACTIONS
Anti-inflammatory, antioxidant, astringent, mild laxative

USED TO TREAT
Colds, influenza, low immunity: tea taken 2–3 times daily is a reviving tonic to the immune system; tablets or capsules taken as directed give the body vitamin C.

Low energy, physical exhaustion: tablets or capsules taken as directed act as a general tonic to boost energy and improve general health.
Fluid retention: tablets or capsules taken as directed help to rid the body of toxins.
Osteo- or rheumatoid arthritis: tablets or capsules taken as directed for a minimum of three months can ease pain and improve movement.

CULINARY USE
Fresh hips can be made into jam, syrup, or wine.

SAFETY INFORMATION
If you are on medication for arthritis, please consult your doctor before taking rose hip as a supplement.

ROSAE (CENTIFOLIA, DAMASCENA, GALLICA)
• ROSE

Rosa centifolia (cabbage rose), *Rosa damascena* (damask rose), and *Rosa gallica* (French rose) are so-called "old fashioned" perfume roses, the ancestors of modern rose hybrids. Typically they have what is called an "untidy habit," meaning they grow in a bushier fashion than the neater modern roses. They can spread up to 6 ft (2 m) in height with trailing prickly stems. Their leaflets are arranged in groups of five or seven, and they produce exquisitely fragrant flowers in a range of shapes and colors: cabbage roses are plump, deep pink blooms; damasks are smaller, simpler flowers in pale pink; and French roses are deep pink or red. These roses need shelter and full sun for at least part of the day, and regular feeding.

Petals from these "old roses" are used to extract essential oil in countries such as Bulgaria, Turkey, and Morocco. Although rose is not used much in herbal medicine any more, rose essential oil has come back into prominence thanks to aromatherapy, where it is used for skin care and to ease emotional stress. It is very expensive to buy neat, but is available already diluted in carrier oils from some essential-oil suppliers as an affordable alternative.

SEE ALSO
Aloe vera, sea buckthorn, evening primrose, lemon verbena, lavender

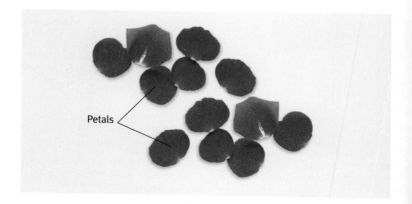

Petals

ROSE

Rosae (centifolia, damascena, gallica)

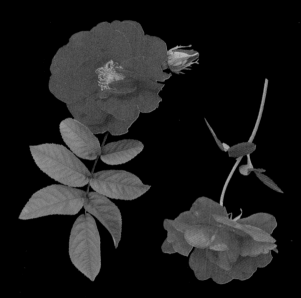

PART OF PLANT USED
Petals

ACTIVE INGREDIENTS
Volatile oil

COMMERCIALLY AVAILABLE AS
Essential oil, rose water, skin-care products

ACTIONS
Astringent, anti-allergic, anti-inflammatory, liver tonic

USED TO TREAT
Burns, sunburn, radiation burns: 2 drops of essential oil in 1 teaspoon (5 ml) of aloe vera gel applied to damaged skin immediately calms angry redness and soothes pain.

Dry or mature skin: 2 drops of essential oil in 1 teaspoon (5 ml) of evening primrose oil massaged into the face and neck morning and night improves skin texture and nourishes the upper skin layers.

Poor liver function: 2 fl oz (60 ml) of pure rose water drunk 2–3 times daily increases the efficiency of the liver.

Emotional stress and anxiety: 2 drops of essential oil added to 1 teaspoon (5 ml) of sunflower carrier massaged into the neck and shoulders eases anxiety and tension.

CULINARY USE
Rose petals can be made into jam.

SAFETY INFORMATION
No issues

ROSMARINUS OFFICINALIS
• ROSEMARY

This evergreen, aromatic shrub grows up to 4 ft (1.2 m) high with woody stems and strongly fragrant, narrow leaves. In early spring it produces pale blue or pink flowers, which are an important source of nourishment for bees. It thrives in sandy, well-drained soil in full sun, and needs shelter in cooler climates. It should be grown from cuttings, ideally, and responds to hard pruning when the bush gets too straggly. The leaves can be used fresh all year round but are most aromatic in July or August when the volatile oil content is highest—this is when they are best picked for drying.

The name "*Rosmarinus*" means "dew of the sea;" this herb originates from the rocky coastlines of the southern Mediterranean. It was probably introduced to Britain by the Romans—in their culture it was considered a symbol of fidelity and was used in bridal wreaths and bouquets. The English playwright William Shakespeare, a keen observer of the plants of his time, mentions rosemary in his play *Hamlet* as being "for remembrance"—today the fragrance is still regarded as an excellent mental tonic.

SEE ALSO
Myrtle, black pepper, cardamom, peppermint, eucalyptus

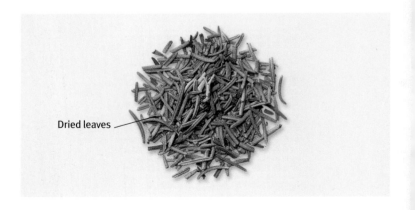

Dried leaves

ROSEMARY

Rosmarinus officinalis

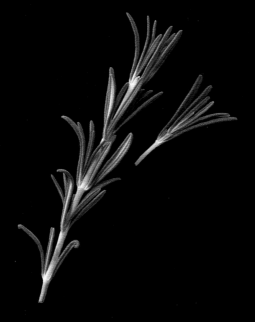

PART OF PLANT USED
Leaves

ACTIVE INGREDIENTS
Organic acids, saponins, tannins, volatile oil

COMMERCIALLY AVAILABLE AS
Fresh and dried herb, essential oil, tablets, tincture, massage balm

ACTIONS
Analgesic, antispasmodic, circulation stimulant, digestive tonic

USED TO TREAT
Muscular aches and pains, sports injuries, rheumatism: 2 drops of essential oil in 1 teaspoon (5 ml) of sunflower oil massaged into affected areas eases pain and stiffness and warms the circulation.
Low physical energy, fatigue: infusion of fresh rosemary leaves drunk 2–3 times daily lifts the spirits and gives a sense of well-being.
Poor concentration: add 2 drops of essential oil to a Kleenex or an electrical diffuser to spread the aroma around you to help mental focus.

CULINARY USE
Rosemary is traditionally used to flavor strong meats such as pork and lamb, as well as in marinades and salad oils.

SAFETY INFORMATION
The essential oil should be avoided by epileptics; also in pregnancy. Culinary use of the herb in pregnancy is safe.

RUBUS IDAEUS
• RASPBERRY

This deciduous shrub has prickly stems up to 5 ft (1.4 m) high, with alternate leaves—deeply veined and toothed at the edges, the upper surfaces are green and hairy and the lower surfaces are white and velvety. It produces white flowers on secondary stems in May or June, followed by the fragrant, red compound berries. Native throughout Europe and parts of Asia, originally the raspberry bush was found growing wild in woodland or on hillsides. If you plant one in your garden it needs full sun and well-drained, slightly acidic soil. It is very fast growing so one shrub is ideal in a small space, while several can make a fruiting hedge. The leaves are best picked for medicinal use just before the flowers open, and used fresh or dried. The fruit is picked when ripe and is best eaten fresh.

Ancient Greek physicians used raspberry fruit and leaves as urinary tonics and decongestants. The botanical name "*Rubus*" means "thorny shrub" and "*idaeus*" is said to refer to Mount Ida in Asia Minor, where raspberries once grew wild in abundance.

SEE ALSO

Marjoram, clary sage, Lady's mantle, fennel, goldenseal

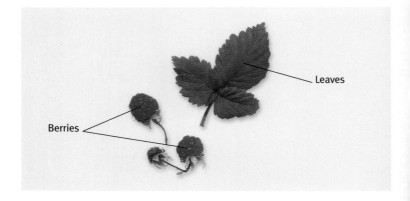

Leaves

Berries

RASPBERRY
Rubus idaeus

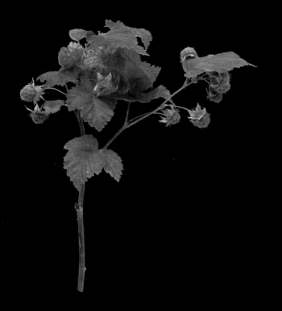

PARTS OF PLANT USED
Leaves, fruit

ACTIVE INGREDIENTS
Organic acids, pectins, tannins, vitamin C

COMMERCIALLY AVAILABLE AS
Tea, tablets, tincture

ACTIONS
Astringent, diuretic, expectorant, galactogogue, uterine tonic

USED TO TREAT
Menstrual pain: infusion of the leaves can be taken 2–3 times daily to ease cramps, also blended with other herbs such as marjoram.
Late pregnancy and childbirth: raspberry-leaf tea can be drunk during the last eight weeks of pregnancy to strengthen the womb and help in labor.
Slow breast milk flow: the tea, taken 2–3 times daily, can improve the production and flow of breast milk.
Sore throats: infusion of the leaves can be used as a gargle to soothe sore throats.

CULINARY USE
Fresh raspberries are rich in vitamin C and make an excellent dessert fruit; they can also be used to make wine or vinegar.

SAFETY INFORMATION
Raspberry-leaf tea should not be taken in early pregnancy because it is a uterine tonic; it can be used later or in labor as above.

RUMEX ACETOSA
• SORREL

Garden sorrel is native to Europe and the British Isles. It is generally found growing wild in pastureland where the soil is rich in iron and nitrogen. It is an example of a nutritious plant that has fallen out of medicinal and culinary use, though at one time it was highly regarded. It is a hardy perennial up to 4 ft (1.2 m) tall, and produces large green leaves with a distinctive point, and tall spikes of reddish brown flowers around midsummer. It is easy to grow from seed, in moist soil, in sun or part shade, and once established it self-seeds quickly. It is best to use the young leaves because they are more tender and contain less oxalic acid.

Various sorrel species were popular in cookery from the 14th century onward; for example, mashed up with vinegar and sugar as an old-fashioned relish with cold meats called "greensauce." In the 16th century sorrel was very popular as a nourishing salad. The 17th-century English herbalist Nicholas Culpeper used it to cool inflammation and fevers, even recommending a poultice made from sorrel to treat plague sores. It was also used to make a green dye for cloth.

SEE ALSO
Mulberry, parsley, celery seed, echinacea, manuka

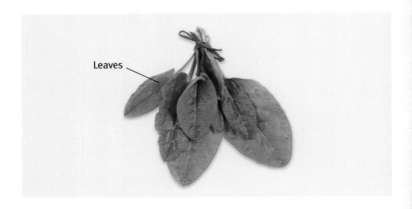

Leaves

SORREL

Rumex acetosa

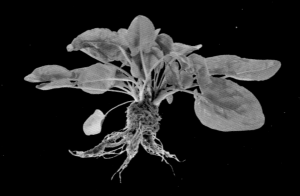

PART OF PLANT USED
Leaves

ACTIVE INGREDIENTS
Oxalic acid, tannins, vitamin C

COMMERCIALLY AVAILABLE AS
Not commercially available, best grown yourself

ACTIONS
Diuretic, detoxifying

USED TO TREAT
Sore throats: an infusion of fresh, young leaves makes a soothing gargle to help sore throats.
Fluid retention: an infusion of fresh, young leaves taken twice daily helps the body detoxify itself.

Fevers: an infusion of fresh, young leaves taken 2–3 times daily helps to cool the body during fever.
Boils, infected cuts and wounds: a handful of young leaves, infused in water and cooled, makes a cleansing wash to treat infected skin.

CULINARY USE
Young, green leaves are used in salad mixtures, or in sorrel soup.

SAFETY INFORMATION
The oxalic acid content of sorrel can interfere with iron absorption, especially if eaten excessively; young leaves should only be used, and sparingly. Do not eat sorrel if you are anemic or pregnant.

SALIX ALBA
• WHITE WILLOW

This large tree, also knows as the European willow, grows up to 80 ft (26 m) in height, with a gray, fissured bark and long sweeping branches with flexible greenish yellow twigs. The pale green leaves are alternate, long, and narrow, with silky white hair on the undersides. White willow is dioecious, meaning both male and female flowers are present on the same tree—seen in the spring as "catkins"—full of pollen and very attractive to bees. It flowers in April and May, sometimes earlier, depending on the temperature. It is native to Europe and the British Isles and grows most successfully beside water or in wet woodland. The bark is used medicinally and can easily be peeled away during the summer—traditionally it was dried and boiled to make tea or decoctions for external use (see page 297).

Young willow twigs have been used in the UK for centuries to make baskets, fencing, and wicker furniture. In the United States, early settlers used the native black willow (*Salix nigra*) in similar ways to the European species. The bark is a natural source of salicin and other salicylic compounds with natural pain-killing and anti-inflammatory effects, traditionally drunk as "willow-bark tea." Today, willow bark has been replaced by synthetic acetosalicylic acid (aspirin), one of the most common pain-killing drugs.

SEE ALSO
Feverfew, centaury, meadowsweet, Devil's claw, lavender

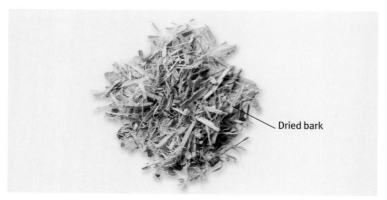

Dried bark

WHITE WILLOW
Salix alba

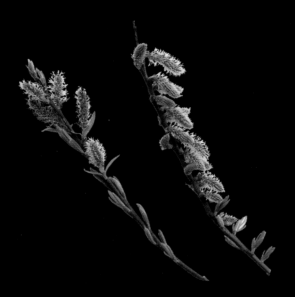

PART OF PLANT USED
Bark

ACTIVE INGREDIENTS
Salicylic compounds including salicin, tannins

COMMERCIALLY AVAILABLE AS
Tea, capsules, tincture

ACTIONS
Analgesic, antipyretic, diaphoretic, antirheumatic

USED TO TREAT
Fevers, high temperatures: tablets, capsules, or tincture taken as directed help reduce temperature and promote sweating to cool the body.
Rheumatism, arthritis: tablets, capsules, or tincture taken as directed ease rheumatic pain and stiffness.
Headaches, migraine: tablets, capsules, or tincture taken as directed ease pain and calm the system.
Indigestion: white willow sometimes occurs in herbal tablet compounds to treat indigestion and diarrhea—take as directed to ease cramps and discomfort.

CULINARY USE
None

SAFETY INFORMATION
No issues; if fever or high temperatures persist, please consult a doctor.

SALVIA OFFICINALIS
• SAGE

This classic herb is evergreen and highly aromatic. It is a shrub that can grow up to 2 ft (60 cm) tall with woody stems and velvety, fragrant gray-green leaves. It produces spikes of purple-blue flowers in early summer, which are very attractive to bees and butterflies. Sage does well in light, well-drained soil in full sun and does not like too much water. It is best started from a plant bought from a garden center, from which cuttings can be taken to produce more bushes. Leaves can be harvested all year round but are most aromatic in August when the volatile oil content is highest—this is the best time to pick them for drying.

The common name "sage" derives from the Latin "*salvere*," meaning to save—since ancient times this herb has been regarded as something of a cure-all. Another old-fashioned name for it is "*Salvia salvatrix*"—"Sage the Savior." The 16th-century herbalist John Gerard regarded it as a tonic to the head and brain, improving alertness and memory, and as a physical tonic to the body, helping weakness and strained muscles.

SEE ALSO
White horehound, myrrh, myrtle, black cohosh, fennel

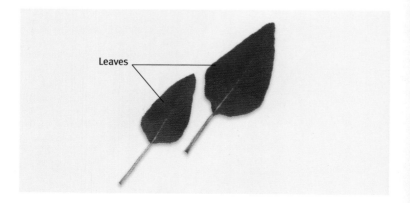

Leaves

SAGE

Salvia officinalis

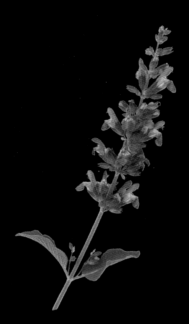

PART OF PLANT USED
Leaves

ACTIVE INGREDIENTS
Bitters, estrogenic compounds, resin, tannins, volatile oil

COMMERCIALLY AVAILABLE AS
Fresh and dried herb, tablets, tincture, tea

ACTIONS
Antiseptic, antispasmodic, diuretic, estrogen balancing

USED TO TREAT
Coughs, chest infections: an infusion of the leaves with an added teaspoon (5 ml) of honey soothes coughs and eases breathing.

Influenza, low immunity: an infusion of the leaves with honey eases aches and strengthens the immune system.
Menopausal problems: tablets or tincture taken as directed help to balance estrogen and reduce symptoms.
Sore throats, ulcers, sore gums: a strong infusion of the leaves makes an antiseptic gargle to clear minor infections in the mouth.

CULINARY USE
Sage has a powerful flavor, good with pork, lamb, and other strong meats, as well as bean and cheese dishes; it also complements cooked apples.

SAFETY INFORMATION
Should not be used medicinally in pregnancy but is safe in culinary use.

SALVIA SCLAREA
• CLARY SAGE

This is one of the largest species of the sage family—clary sage grows
to an impressive 4ft (1.2 m) height. Originally native to southern Europe,
particularly France and Italy, it was introduced to Britain in the 16th
century. It has very large, velvety, pointed leaves and produces tall
spikes of pinkish blue flowers in late summer. The whole plant has a very
distinctive fragrance—musky, nutty, and pungent. It likes moist, fertile
soil in full sun and can be grown from seed sown in the spring. It dies off
in the second year, but will have produced plenty of seeds for re-sowing.
The leaves can be used throughout the season, the flowering tops are
harvested in early summer for essential-oil production, and the seeds can
be collected in late summer.

An old French name for this herb is "*toute bonne*," meaning "all good," and
the common name "clary" is a corruption of "clear eye," referring to an ancient
use of the herb as a soothing eyewash. In the 19th century clary sage was
used as an alternative to hops, making very heady beers thanks to the volatile
oil content. Today, commercially extracted clary sage essential oil is used in
aromatherapy as a hormone balancing remedy.

SEE ALSO

Marjoram, Lady's mantle, agnus castus, black cohosh, raspberry

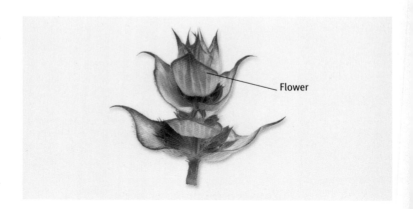

Flower

CLARY SAGE

Salvia sclarea

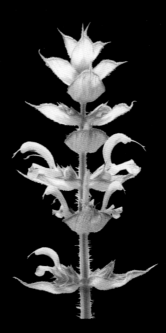

PART OF PLANT USED
Flowering tops

ACTIVE INGREDIENTS
Bitters, tannins, volatile oil

COMMERCIALLY AVAILABLE AS
Essential oil

ACTIONS
Antispasmodic, hormone balancing, uterine tonic, circulation stimulating

USED TO TREAT
PMS, menstrual cramps: 2 drops of essential oil in a warm evening bathtub just before the onset of menstruation helps raise energy levels and ease PMS discomfort.
Menopausal problems: 2 drops of essential oil in 1 teaspoon (5 ml) of sunflower oil can be massaged into the chest and abdomen as needed to help balance menopausal hormone fluctuations.
Late pregnancy or labor: 1 drop of essential oil in 1 teaspoon (5 ml) of sunflower oil (note the low amount) can be massaged daily into the abdomen and lower back in the last month of pregnancy and during labor.

CULINARY USE
None

SAFETY INFORMATION
Clary sage essential oil should not be used in massage or bathtubs for the first eight months of pregnancy because of its uterine tonic effect.

SAMBUCUS NIGRA
• ELDER

A vigorous shrub still found growing wild all over Europe and the British Isles in woodland, along riverbanks, and on waste ground, elder grows up to 30 ft (10 m) in height. It has dull green leaves, and produces flat heads of hundreds of tiny cream-colored flowers in early summer. These become clusters of small, black, shiny berries in late summer or early fall. Harvest the flowers early but leave enough to produce berries later. Although some ornamental elder varieties exist, only the wild species is of medicinal value. It is so vigorous that simply breaking twigs off an existing shrub and pushing them into soil may actually produce new plants. Elder requires moist, well-drained soil, in sun or partial shade.

The Romans called this tree "*Sambucus*," which is part of the botanical name. "*Nigra*" means "black," referring to the color of the berries. The common name "elder" comes from the Anglo-Saxon "*aeld*," meaning "fire," because the twigs are hollow and were used in ancient times to blow sparks into flame. Elder is widely associated with folklore: in northern Europe superstition still forbids cutting the branches or wood without first asking permission of the "*Hlyde-Moer*"—the "elder mother" spirit who lives in the tree.

SEE ALSO

Yarrow, peppermint, eucalyptus, eyebright, Roman camomile

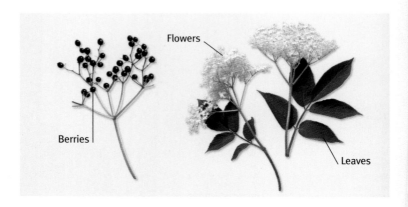

Flowers

Berries

Leaves

ELDER
Sambucus nigra

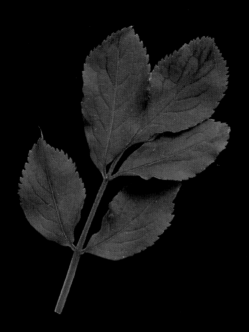

PARTS OF PLANT USED
Flowers, berries

ACTIVE INGREDIENTS
Flowers—glycosides, organic acids, mucilage, tannins; berries—vitamin C

COMMERCIALLY AVAILABLE AS
Tea, cough medicine, tablets, tincture

ACTIONS ·
Anti-inflammatory, diaphoretic, expectorant

USED TO TREAT
Coughs, colds, influenza: an infusion of equal parts of elder flower, yarrow (see pages 22–3), and peppermint (see pages 172–3) taken 2–3 times daily is a standard remedy for cold and flu symptoms; syrup or medicine made from the berries, taken as directed, acts as a respiratory tonic and is very palatable to children.
Hay fever: tablets, capsules, or tincture taken as directed can help build resistance to allergies.
Sore or inflamed skin: infusion of fresh flowers, cooled, applied to sore or reddened skin has an anti-inflammatory effect.

CULINARY USE
Elder flowers can be fried in batter as a delicate summer treat; the berries can be made into wine.

SAFETY INFORMATION
Elder leaves have powerful purgative effects and should not be taken internally.

SAPONARIA OFFICINALIS
• SOAPWORT

A tall, perennial herb, soapwort grows from a tough, orange-colored, creeping root system. It has erect stems growing up to 5 ft (1.5 m) in height, covered with tiny, silky hairs. The leaves are arranged opposite each other, and are long and lance-shaped, tapering to a graceful point, each with three deep veins. The flowers are pale pink, opening in clusters. It thrives in very moist soils, and in the wild it is usually found in ditches or by streams. It can easily be grown from seed and spreads quickly. The roots are the active medicinal part, and these should be harvested (from plants that are a minimum of two years old), cleaned, and dried for storage.

Native all over Europe and the British Isles, soapwort has been cultivated for centuries. Before the widespread use and availability of soap, soaking the roots released their high quantities of natural saponins, causing a foaming effect—the botanical name "*Saponaria*" is from the Latin "*sapo*" for "soap." Soapwort was used to wash clothing, especially items made of wool or silk, and has also been valued for centuries as a skin cleansing and healing agent because of its externally anti-inflammatory effects. Internally, however, it has an extremely powerful purgative effect so soapwort should only be taken under professional guidance.

SEE ALSO
Echinacea, tea tree, calendula, evening primrose, heather

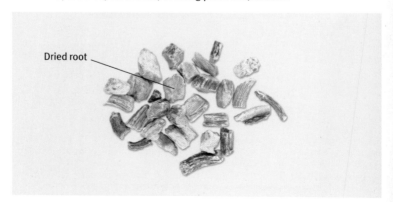

Dried root

SOAPWORT

Saponaria officinalis

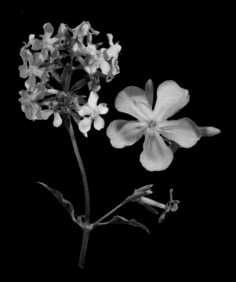

PART OF PLANT USED
Roots

ACTIVE INGREDIENTS
Flavonoids, saponins, sugar

COMMERCIALLY AVAILABLE AS
Dried root, only available from
professional herbalists

ACTIONS
Anti-inflammatory, expectorant, diuretic,
laxative

USED TO TREAT
Boils, acne: a decoction of the root (see
page 297) applied to affected areas
2–3 times daily reduces inflammation,
cleanses the tissues, and speeds healing.
Eczema, psoriasis: a decoction as
above applied to affected areas 2–3
times daily soothes irritation and sore,
reddened skin.
Gout, rheumatism: a decoction as above,
prepared and added to a warm bath,
soothes pain and stiffness and helps
reduce inflammation.

CULINARY USE
None

SAFETY INFORMATION
Internal use of soapwort should only be
under professional guidance because
large doses can irritate the lining of the
digestive and respiratory tracts.

SATUREIA HORTENSIS
• SAVORY

This small, bushy, annual herb, also called summer savory, produces erect, woody stems up to 15 in (38 cm) tall, and small, lance-shaped, dark green aromatic leaves, as well as tiny white flowers in high summer. It needs well-drained soil in full sun and can be planted in pots. If planted between rows of beans, savory will help to keep away black fly and other pests, because the whole plant has a strong aroma. Savory can be grown from seed in the garden in late spring, once frosts are over. Harvest the leaves— the medicinal part—in August, when they are most aromatic, because the volatile oil content is high.

The botanical name "*Satureia*" was first used by the Roman writer Pliny in the 1st century CE, and is thought to be linked to the notion of the satyr, a mythical figure that was half-man, half-goat, because the herb was considered to be an aphrodisiac. Virgil, another famous Roman writer, praised the fragrance of the plant. Savory leaves have a peppery taste, and they were used in Roman meat recipes as a pungent seasoning before the arrival of spices. The 17th-century English herbalist Nicholas Culpeper used a syrup made with the leaves as a winter remedy for coughs and phlegm.

SEE ALSO
Peppermint, spearmint, myrtle, rosemary, basil

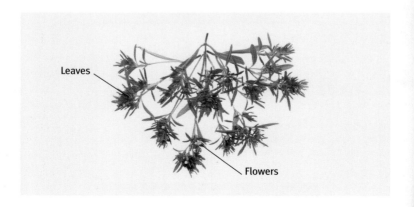

Leaves

Flowers

SAVORY

Satureia hortensis

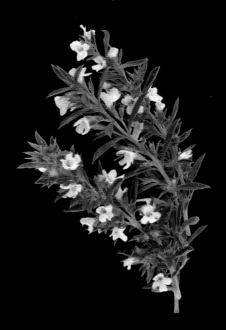

PART OF PLANT USED
Leaves

ACTIVE INGREDIENTS
Mucilage, resins, tannins, volatile oil

COMMERCIALLY AVAILABLE AS
Dried herb, essential oil

ACTIONS
Antispasmodic, astringent, carminative, digestive tonic, expectorant, emmenagogue

USED TO TREAT
Indigestion, gas, bloating: an infusion of fresh savory leaves taken after meals has a calming effect on digestion and eases the pressure of gas in the gut.
Chesty coughs, catarrh: an infusion of fresh savory leaves with a teaspoon (5 ml) of honey, taken 2–3 times daily, helps soothe chesty coughs and loosen catarrh.
Bee and wasp stings: fresh savory leaves rubbed onto stings help to reduce pain and inflammation.

CULINARY USE
Cooking savory leaves with beans improves their flavor and helps prevent gas. Savory also peps up vegetarian nut roasts or patés, and egg dishes.

SAFETY INFORMATION
The essential oil should not be used in pregnancy because it can stimulate menstrual bleeding.

SCUTELLARIA LATERIFOLIA
• SKULLCAP

Skullcap is native to North America, growing in profusion in wet locations throughout Canada and the north and eastern regions of the United States. Skullcap thrives in well-drained soil in full sunlight. It is a perennial plant, with a fibrous, yellow root system and a branching stem up to 4 ft (1.2 m) tall. It has heart-shaped leaves with scalloped edges. Its flowers are pale blue or sometimes light purple in color, and grow from the axils, where the leaf stems join the main stem. Flowering occurs between May and August. For medicinal purposes the flowering tops are collected just before the plant comes into full bloom, and are then carefully dried before storage.

Many species of skullcap exist across the world, from North America, where there are at least 90 types, to Europe and Asia. The Cherokee and other Native American tribes used skullcap extensively as a herb for menstrual problems and to aid recovery from childbirth, while in Europe it was used traditionally to help epilepsy and troubles of the nervous system. Today the plant is still mostly collected from the wild, as cultivation attempts have proved ineffective. This species, *Scutellaria laterifolia*, is one of the most important for medicinal purposes, and in Georgia research is being conducted into methods of cultivation to help protect wild species from over-harvesting.

SEE ALSO
Passion flower, valerian, raspberry leaf, wild yam, meadowsweet

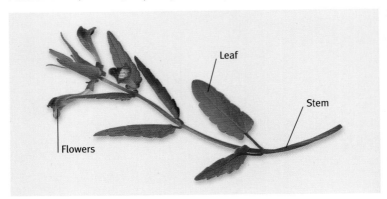

Leaf

Stem

Flowers

SKULLCAP

Scutellaria laterifolia

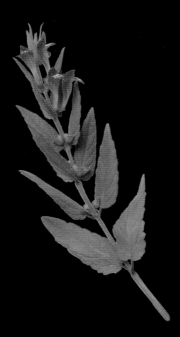

PART OF PLANT USED
Flowering tops

ACTIVE INGREDIENTS
Bitters, flavonoid glycosides, tannins, volatile oil

COMMERCIALLY AVAILABLE AS
Tea, tablets, capsules, tincture

ACTIONS
Antidepressant, nerve tonic

USED TO TREAT
Insomnia, emotional stress: tablets, capsules, or tincture taken as directed ease pain and relax the nervous system, relieving anxiety and tension.
Irregular periods, PMS: tablets, capsules, or tincture taken as directed relieve stress-related PMS and menstrual difficulties.
Stress-related headaches, migraine: tablets, capsules, or tincture taken as directed ease pain and relieve symptoms made worse by emotional stress.

CULINARY USE
None

SAFETY INFORMATION
If you are on conventional medication for depression or pain relief, consult a doctor or professional herbalist before using skullcap.

SERENOA SERRULATA
• SAW PALMETTO

This small palm tree is native to the West Indies and the Atlantic coast of the United States, namely South Carolina, Georgia, coastal Alabama, and, most importantly, Florida. It grows in profusion in thickets called "palmetto scrub," covering areas totalling millions of acres. A tropical tree, it thrives in areas of high humidity and heat; its leaves are tough and toothed, easily able to tear clothing or skin, as suggested by the common name "saw." Its berries, the medicinal part, ripen between August and September and have to be picked by hand for production of the herbal supplement, before being cleaned and dried before processing.

In the United States, saw palmetto was first recognized as a potent remedy for the health of the prostate and male sexual organs in the 19th and early 20th centuries. Widespread clinical research throughout Europe, particularly in France, Great Britain, and Germany, has highlighted the benefits of saw palmetto to relieve the symptoms of benign prostatic hyperplasia (BPH) — when the prostate gland enlarges and causes urinary problems in older men. Since as many as one in three men may be affected by BPH, the availability of an herbal alternative to medication is attractive. However, the condition should be monitored by a doctor and simple self-medication is not advised.

SEE ALSO
Pasque flower, ginseng, myrtle, myrrh, white horehound

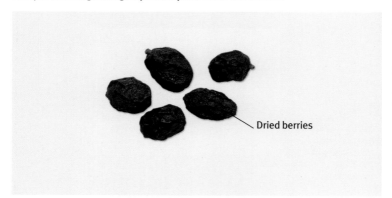

Dried berries

SAW PALMETTO
Serenoa serrulata

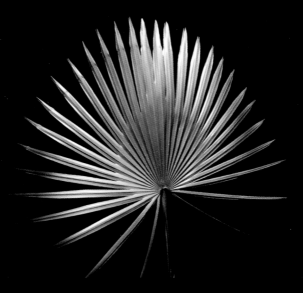

PART OF PLANT USED
Berries

ACTIVE INGREDIENTS
Resin, saponins, tannins, volatile oil

COMMERCIALLY AVAILABLE AS
Capsules, tablets, tincture

ACTIONS
Anti-inflammatory, antispasmodic, expectorant, sexual tonic, sedative

USED TO TREAT
Benign prostatic hyperplasia (BPH): tablets, capsules, or tincture taken as directed may have a tonic effect on the male sexual organs, including the prostate gland.
Low libido, impotence: tablets, capsules, or tincture taken as directed act as a tonic to the male sexual organs, as well as easing nervous stress.
Colds, bronchitis: tablets, capsules, or tincture taken as directed have an expectorant effect on the system, easing coughs and helping to expel mucus.

CULINARY USE
None

SAFETY INFORMATION
Any difficulties with urination or discomfort should be reported to a doctor. If you are already taking medication, especially anticoagulant drugs, seek medical advice before any use of saw palmetto.

SILYBUM MARIANUM
• MILK THISTLE

This tall spiny plant grows up to 2 ft (60 cm) high, with an erect, furrowed stem. The leaves are alternate, with sharp, thorny edges—the lower ones are smaller and the higher ones spread out more widely around the stem. The flower is a disc of purple, tubular petals, forming a typical thistle-like head, sitting on a circular array of spines. The seeds—the medicinal part of the plant—are oval-shaped and black. Other common names for this plant are elephant thistle or ivory thistle. Originally native to the southern Mediterranean, North Africa, and the Middle East, milk thistle thrives in a tough, arid environment with plenty of sun. It is now cultivated for its medicinal value all over Europe.

As the name suggests, one old-fashioned use for the seeds was to promote milk in nursing mothers, although this property has never been borne out scientifically. The modern use for milk thistle is as a liver tonic because of the strong concentration of bitter compounds it contains. Its active ingredient is called silymarin, and it is reputed to help to tone and regenerate the liver.

SEE ALSO:
Yellow gentian, centaury, fennel, grapefruit, parsley

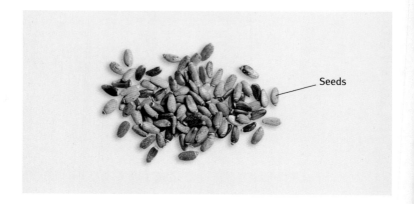

Seeds

MILK THISTLE

Silybum marianum

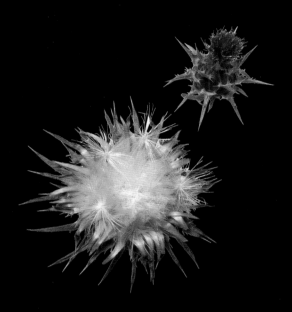

PART OF PLANT USED
Seeds

ACTIVE INGREDIENTS
Bitters, fatty oil, protein, flavones (silymarin), volatile oil

COMMERICALLY AVAILABLE AS
Capsules, tablets, tincture

ACTIONS
Digestive and liver tonic, cholagogue/chloretic (controlling the production and flow of bile)

USED TO TREAT
Sluggish digestion, especially of fatty foods: tablets, capsules, or tincture taken as directed improve the liver's ability to digest fats.

Poor liver function: tablets, capsules, or tincture taken as directed strengthen and tone the liver to improve its function.
Liver damage (from alcohol or drug use): tablets, capsules, or tincture taken as directed may help support the liver through detoxification.

CULINARY USE
None, although apparently young leaves and shoots used to be boiled and eaten as a vegetable.

SAFETY INFORMATION
If you are on medication for the liver or are seeking support for tobacco withdrawal or drug rehabilitation, you should do so under medical guidance and seek professional advice about taking milk thistle.

SOLIDAGO VIRGAUREA
• GOLDENROD

A perennial herb that can grow up to 3 ft (1 m) tall, goldenrod has an erect and downy stem, sometimes branching at the top. It produces long, narrow, lance-shaped leaves tapering to a point, becoming narrower and shorter as the flowering stem takes shape. Its flowers are small and yellow and arranged in groups of ten or so at the end of a stalk. The related Canadian goldenrod (*Solidago canadiensis*) looks very similar and has parallel medicinal uses. Goldenrod thrives in dry woodland and grassland, and often arrives in gardens by itself as a wild plant. The flowering tops are used medicinally, harvested as the flowers come into bloom.

This herb has been used for hundreds of years to treat kidney and bladder disorders; it helps to dissolve what used to be called "gravel"—that is, fragments of kidney stones in the urine. The 17th-century English herbalist Nicholas Culpeper regarded it as one of the most beneficially cleansing herbal teas. Externally, it has always been considered a very effective wound-healing herb, especially good for ulcers, eczema, and skin that is slow to heal.

SEE ALSO

Bearberry/uva ursi, wild strawberry, saw palmetto, German camomile, yarrow

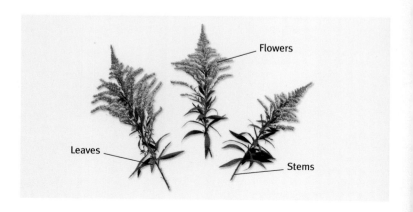

Flowers

Leaves

Stems

GOLDENROD

Solidago virgaurea

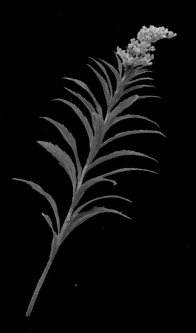

PART OF PLANT USED
Flowering tops

ACTIVE INGREDIENTS
Bitters, flavonoids, saponins, tannins, volatile oil

COMMERCIALLY AVAILABLE AS
Capsules, tea, tincture

ACTIONS
Anti-inflammatory, astringent, diuretic, vulnerary

USED TO TREAT
Urinary-tract and kidney infections: capsules or tincture taken as directed, or tea taken 2–3 times daily, ease the flow of urine and soothes irritation (if symptoms persist seek medical advice).

Prostate and kidney problems: capsules or tincture taken as directed strengthen the prostate and urinary organs.
Skin ulcers, eczema, slow healing wounds: goldenrod ointment applied 2–3 times daily encourages skin healing.
Heavy menstrual bleeding: goldenrod tea has an ancient reputation as a treatment for excess menstruation; take it twice a day for the week up to the onset of a period.

CULINARY USE
None

SAFETY INFORMATION
If you are on medication for kidney or urinary conditions or are concerned that these may be a problem, seek medical guidance before using goldenrod.

STACHYS OFFICINALIS
• WOOD BETONY

This perennial herb grows from a thick, woody root up to heights of 2 ft (60 cm). Most of its leaves are arranged in a rosette around its base, and they are oval, wrinkled, and toothed at the edges. Its stem is vertical and four-sided, mostly without branches. At the tip of each stem the reddish flowers are arranged in clusters, called "whorls," forming a terminal spike. Betony is native all over Europe and the British Isles, where it thrives in woodland, hedgerows, and on open moorland. With many of these habitats now under threat, picking the wild herb may be prohibited in some areas, although some seed suppliers are beginning to sell wild flower species, to enable them to be planted in gardens for conservation. The flowering tops are the medicinal part of the plant, collected for drying just as the blooms appear.

Betony takes its common name from its original Latin name "*vetonica*," which became "*betonica*" over time (it is sometimes referred to botanically as "*Betonica officinalis*"). For hundreds of years it was considered something of a cure-all, and also a plant with magical powers. However, in modern herbal medicine, it has largely fallen out of common use, though it remains popular in France as a liver and gall-bladder tonic.

SEE ALSO:
Witch hazel, arnica, pasque flower, meadowsweet, yellow gentian

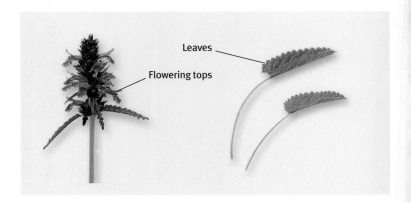

Leaves

Flowering tops

WOOD BETONY

Stachys officinalis

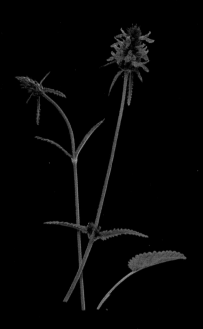

PART OF PLANT USED
Flowering tops

ACTIVE INGREDIENTS
Alkaloids, saponins, tannins

COMMERCIALLY AVAILABLE AS
Dried herb (from specialist suppliers only)

ACTIONS
Anti-inflammatory, antiseptic, digestive and liver tonic, sedative, vulnerary

USED TO TREAT
Cuts, wounds, bruises: a strong infusion of the flowering tops, cooled, applied to damaged areas, helps to clean away dirt and reduce swelling; it can also be applied as a cold compress to bruises.
Headaches, migraines: drink an infusion of the flowering tops twice daily to help calm the nervous system and reduce stress.
Sluggish digestion: an infusion taken 2–3 times daily after meals acts as a tonic to the liver to help digest heavy foods.

CULINARY USE
None

SAFETY INFORMATION
In large doses betony can be very purgative, causing severe diarrhea—do not take more than the amounts stated above, and not for prolonged periods.

SYMPHYTUM OFFICINALE
• COMFREY

A perennial herb that grows vigorously, comfrey has a thick, dark-colored root system. Above ground, it reaches up to 4 ft (1.2 m) in height and about 3 ft (1 m) in width. Its foliage is made up of very large, fleshy, hairy leaves, and small, violet or pink flowers appear in early summer on separate stalks. Comfrey thrives in damp soil and partially shady conditions. It can be dug up in the spring and roots separated into several clumps for replanting to help it spread. Young leaves are used medicinally to make ointment or macerated oil (see page 297), and the roots are made into a tincture.

Native throughout Europe, comfrey has been cultivated for centuries because of its healing effects. Another old name for comfrey is "knitbone," showing its long-established reputation for healing broken bones. In recent times, scientific concerns have been raised about some of the alkaloid ingredients in comfrey and possible side-effects on the liver, leading to its internal use being banned in Great Britain since 2002. Other countries, such as Australia, will only allow its internal use as a homeopathic remedy. Ointments and massage oils containing comfrey are still readily available for external use.

SEE ALSO
Arnica, aloe vera, rose, sea buckthorn, horse chestnut

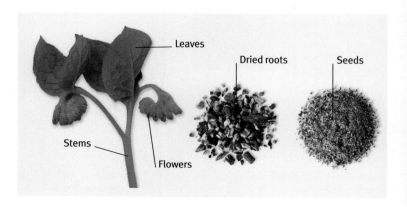

Leaves

Dried roots

Seeds

Stems

Flowers

COMFREY

Symphytum officinale

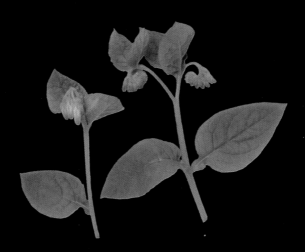

PARTS OF PLANT USED
Leaves, roots

ACTIVE INGREDIENTS
Allantoin, alkaloids, mucilage, tannin, volatile oil

COMMERCIALLY AVAILABLE AS
Ointment, massage oil, cream, tincture

ACTIONS
Anti-inflammatory, antiseptic, emollient

USED TO TREAT
Bruises, sprains: an infusion of comfrey leaves, cooled, can be applied to bruises or sprains as a cold compress to reduce swelling.
Broken bones: a cold comfrey infusion compress reduces swelling and pain.

Burns: ointment of comfrey or an infusion of the leaves, cooled, applied to the skin reduces inflammation.
Varicose veins: ointment applied to varicose veins 2–3 times daily reduces inflammation and eases aching legs.

CULINARY USE
None

SAFETY INFORMATION
Internal use is banned in many countries, while others allow it only in homeopathic doses. Some herbalists maintain comfrey should not be used on open cuts or wounds because of the alkaloid content.

TABEBUIA AVELLANEDAE
• PAU D'ARCO

This large and beautiful tree is native to the Amazon rainforest and tropical zones of South America. It grows up to 100 ft (30 m) tall and its trunk can be up to 10 ft (3 m) wide. It produces dramatic purple flowers. The inner bark of the tree is the active medicinal part, harvested for centuries by native people across its indigenous habitat, and used to treat a huge variety of ailments, such as respiratory problems, fungal infections, arthritic conditions, snake and insect bites, skin problems, and even tumors. Many local names given to the tree by Amazon tribes praise its strength and vitality, while its wood is revered as a material to make bows and weapons.

Pau d'arco gained popularity in Western herbal practice in the 1950s and 1960s, when the bark was analyzed and found to contain compounds with potential antitumoral effects. However, continued investigations since the 1970s have highlighted side-effects from high doses taken internally, and its antitumoral effects have been questioned. The bark has shown strong antimicrobial effects against viruses, parasites, and yeasts such as *Candida albicans*. Though many scientists still remain skeptical about the effects of pau d'arco, the tea can be drunk safely as an immune-enhancing tonic, and capsules, tablets, or tincture are readily available.

SEE ALSO
Tea tree, manuka, garlic, echinacea, fennel

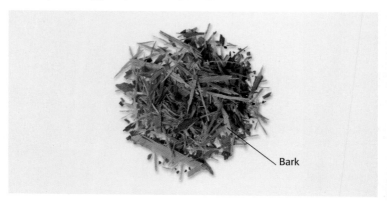

Bark

PAU D'ARCO
Tabebuia avellanedae

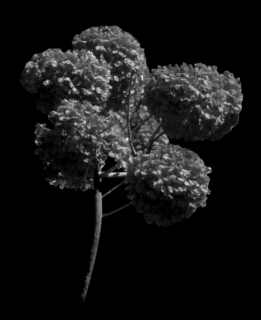

PART OF PLANT USED
Inner bark

ACTIVE INGREDIENTS
Flavonoids, quinoids

COMMERCIALLY AVAILABLE AS
Tea, capsules, tablets, tincture

ACTIONS
Antimicrobial, antifungal, antiviral, antitumoral (potential)

USED TO TREAT
Influenza, colds: tea, tablets, capsules, or tincture taken as directed stimulate the immune system to fight infection.
Yeast infections (candida): a strong infusion of the bark can be used as a douche treatment for vaginal thrush; tablets, capsules, or tincture can be taken as directed for a preventive effect.
Urinary tract infections: tablets, capsules, or tincture taken as directed help to rid the urinary system of bacteria.

CULINARY USE
None

SAFETY INFORMATION
Large internal doses can cause nausea and vomiting. Prolonged use of capsules, tablets, or tincture should be taken under professional supervision. Avoid during pregnancy because some of its constituents are abortifacient.

TANACETUM PARTHENICUM
• FEVERFEW

This bushy, hardy perennial grows up to 3 ft (1 m) tall, with divided, silky, dark green, aromatic leaves. The small flowers have white petals and yellow centers. Originally native to southeastern Europe and Asia Minor, it has spread via the Mediterranean to many other parts of the world, mostly through cultivation. Although some ornamental varieties exist, such as "*Aureum*" with golden leaves, these do not have medicinal properties— only the original species is useful. Feverfew grows in any type of soil, even surviving drought. Seeds can be planted in spring, or cuttings taken from mature plants. The leaves and flowers can be used fresh or picked in high summer, before being carefully dried and stored.

The common name feverfew may come from the Latin "*febris*," meaning fever, and "*fugure*," meaning to chase away; this has always been one of its main uses. The 17th-century English herbalist Nicholas Culpeper prized it as a treatment for headaches and many female disorders, such as menstrual irregularity, and depression. Modern research since the 1970s has highlighted constituents in feverfew leaves that may cause dilation of peripheral blood vessels, explaining why the plant helps conditions such as migraine, where spasmodic pain occurs because of circulation restriction.

SEE ALSO
Valerian, white willow, rose hip, oat, hops

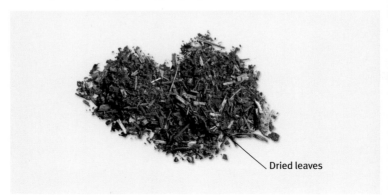

Dried leaves

FEVERFEW
Tanacetum parthenicum

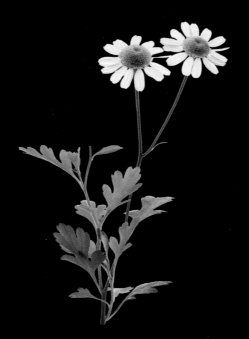

PART OF PLANT USED
Leaves

ACTIVE INGREDIENTS
Bitters, mucilage, tannins,
volatile oil

COMMERCIALLY AVAILABLE AS
Tablets, tincture

ACTIONS
Analgesic, antispasmodic, sedative

USED TO TREAT
Migraines, headaches: an infusion of
fresh leaves, or tablets or tincture taken
as directed ease spasmodic pain.
Menstrual pain: tablets or tincture taken
as directed, particularly in the week
prior to onset of the period, help to ease
cramps and premenstrual discomfort.
Arthritis: an infusion taken as above, or
tablets or tincture taken as directed ease
spasmodic pain and discomfort.
Insomnia due to stress: an infusion or
tablets or tincture taken as directed,
especially in the evening, help to relax
the mind and prepare for sleep.

CULINARY USE
None

SAFETY INFORMATION
Do not take feverfew if you are on
medication for migraine or arthritis, or
if you are taking anticoagulant drugs
such as Warfarin. Do not exceed stated
doses—this can lead to mouth ulcers.

TARAXACUM OFFICINALE
• DANDELION

This familiar plant needs little introduction — gardeners are all too familiar with it as a weed. However, it is an example of a humble plant that was far more respected in the past than it is now. It grows on a stout tap root, producing lush, green leaves on stalks with a milky discharge when broken; its single flower stalk matures into a golden yellow daisy-like head, followed by spherical fluffy seed heads that spread themselves with effortless efficiency. The root is the most important medicinal part, harvested mainly in the fall when the bitter compounds are at their highest levels, and then dried.

The name "*Taraxacum*" seems to be derived from two Greek words: "*taraxos*," meaning disorder and "*akos*," meaning remedy. Since ancient Greek times, this plant has been valued for its internally cleansing and diuretic effects. The common name is from the French "*dent de lion*," meaning "lion's teeth," because of the ragged shape of the leaves. In 19th-century Britain dandelion leaves were used to make beer, as well as a traditional cordial, "dandelion and burdock." Dandelion wine was made from the flowers.

SEE ALSO
Lemon verbena, Devil's claw, celery seed, bearberry/uva ursi, juniper

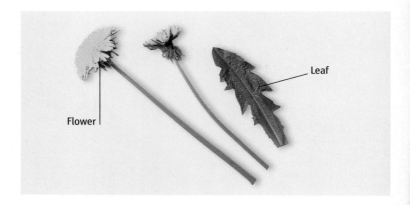

Leaf

Flower

DANDELION

Taraxacum officinale

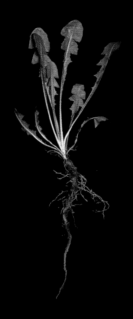

PART OF PLANT USED
Roots, leaves

ACTIVE INGREDIENTS
Bitters, glycosides, resin, sterols, volatile oil

COMMERCIALLY AVAILABLE AS
Tea, capsules, tincture, coffee substitute

ACTIONS
Digestive tonic, diuretic, mild laxative, liver tonic

USED TO TREAT
Indigestion, sluggish digestion, constipation: tea, or tablets or tincture taken as directed, especially after heavy meals, act as a bitter tonic and mild laxative, improving digestion.

Fluid retention, urinary infections: tea, or capsules or tincture taken as directed improve the flow of urine and enhance kidney function.
Rheumatism: dandelion cleanses the blood and tissues and is a useful detoxifying remedy; try eating fresh leaves in salads, or take capsules or tincture as directed.

CULINARY USE
Young leaves can be added to salads; roasted ground dried root makes a pleasant coffee substitute.

SAFETY INFORMATION
Do not use dandelion medicinally if you are taking diuretic medication, or if you have a medically diagnosed kidney problem—seek medical advice first.

THYMUS VULGARIS
• THYME

A low-growing perennial up to 18 in (45 cm) tall, thyme has woody stems and tiny, twig-like branches forming a dense mat of tiny, dark green, aromatic leaves. Spikes of pinkish flowers occur in high summer. The whole plant is very attractive to bees, butterflies, and other beneficial insects. There are many varieties—for example, *Thymus serpyllum* and *Thymus pulegoides* have larger, more oval leaves, while *Thymus x citriodorus* is lemon-scented. It is best to grow thyme plants from a reputable supplier to get the right species—once established, cuttings can be taken from a parent plant. All thyme needs well-drained, preferably sandy soil, with as much sun and heat as possible. Native to the southern Mediterranean region, plants also grow well in rock gardens and tolerate drought. Although the leaves can be harvested all year round, the flavor is best in high summer when the volatile-oil content is highest.

The ancient Greeks burned thyme as a purifying incense to cleanse temples and homes. The name thyme may be linked to the Greek word "*thumus*," meaning courage—the powerful aroma has long been appreciated for its positive effects on the mind. Roman writers praised thyme as a fumigator and antiseptic. The plant is likely to have been introduced into Britain by the Romans.

SEE ALSO

Goldenseal, raspberry leaf, white horehound, elder, cayenne

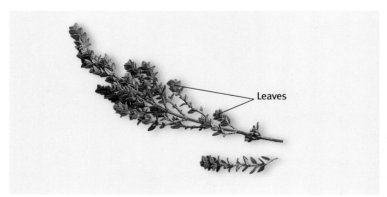

Leaves

THYME

Thymus vulgaris

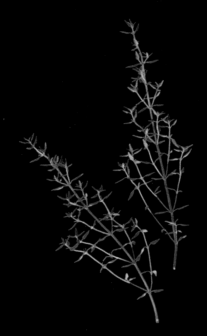

PART OF PLANT USED
Leaves

ACTIVE INGREDIENTS
Bitters, flavonoids, saponins, tannins, volatile oil

COMMERCIALLY AVAILABLE AS
Fresh and dried herb, capsules, lozenges, liniment, cough medicine

ACTIONS
Antimicrobial, antiseptic, expectorant, vulnerary

USED TO TREAT
Sore throats, hoarseness of voice: lozenges can be sucked, or an infusion of fresh leaves, cooled, can be used as a gargle to soothe and fight infection.

Coughs: cough medicine taken as directed, or a warm infusion of fresh leaves with a teaspoon of honey eases spasmodic coughs.
Poor circulation, muscular aches and pains: liniment applied to aching muscles 2–3 times daily warms and improves circulation.

CULINARY USE
Add to meat or fish dishes, and to root vegetables such as carrots; macerate in herbal vinegars and oils.

SAFETY INFORMATION
Thyme is not advised medicinally in pregnancy because it can stimulate menstruation. Culinary use is safe.

TILIA CORDATA
• LIME FLOWER

This species, also commonly called the linden tree, can grow to more than 100 ft (30 m) in height, with strong, downward-curving branches and a gray bark. Its foliage is made up of alternate leaves, dark green above and gray-green below, with an overall heart-shape and serrated edges. The blooms—known as "lime flowers" or "linden blossom"—are tiny, highly fragrant yellowish white clusters, very attractive to bees. Lime flower honey is also beautifully scented and delicious, and a single tree can yield as much as 10 lb (4.5 kg). Native all over central and southern Europe, the whole tree is heavily fragrant in midsummer, when the flowers can be collected for drying.

The inner wood of the lime tree is extremely flexible and resilient; ancient Anglo-Saxon weapon makers relied on it for the construction of their rounded shields. The inner, fibrous bark was also used for rope making and the weaving of mats. The name "linden" is from the Anglo-Saxon word "*lind*"—their ancient name for the tree. The wood also lends itself to intricate carving, and was used to create sculptures and decorative screens in cathedrals. In Europe, the trees are often planted as decorative features along boulevards or in parks.

SEE ALSO
Echinacea, elder, bitter orange, spearmint, melissa

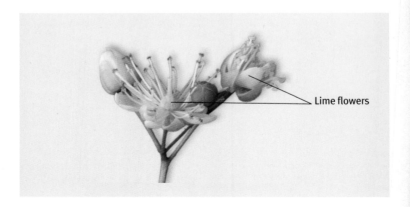
Lime flowers

250

LIME FLOWER

Tilia cordata

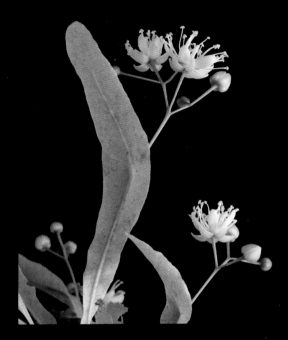

PART OF PLANT USED
Flowers

ACTIVE INGREDIENTS
Flavonoid glycosides, mucilage, saponins, sugar, tannins, volatile oil

COMMERCIALLY AVAILABLE AS
Tea, tablets, capsules; also as an "absolute" (an aromatic extract produced by soaking the flowers in solvent) from aromatherapy suppliers and perfumeries

ACTIONS
Antispasmodic, diaphoretic, diuretic, sedative

USED TO TREAT
Fevers, chills, influenza: tea taken 3–4 times daily encourages sweating and helps the body to cope with the progress of a viral episode.
Stress-related indigestion: tea taken after meals, or tablets or capsules as directed help reduce anxiety and ease digestive processes.
Insomnia, nervous stress: tea taken at night relaxes the mind and improves sleep quality; tablets or capsules taken over a longer period help to calm mental tension. A handful of fresh flowers added to an evening bath also promotes a feeling of deep relaxation.

CULINARY USE
None

SAFETY INFORMATION
No issues

TRIFOLIUM PRAETENSE
• RED CLOVER

This short-lived, perennial plant grows up to 2 ft (60 cm) tall, and forms mats of foliage among grasses. Its soft, green leaves are trifoliate and its composite flowers are deep pink, with hundreds of tiny blooms packed into one flowerhead. Red clover needs moist, well-drained soil, full sun, and can easily be grown from seed. The flowers are the active medicinal part, and should be harvested for drying when they are in full bloom, which can be any time from May through to September. At the end of the growing season plants can be dug back into the ground as "green manure" to add nutrients to the soil.

Originally native to Europe, growing wild in pastures, on hillsides, and in meadows, red clover has been cultivated as animal fodder since prehistoric times. The common name "clover" comes from the Anglo-Saxon name for the plant, "*claefre*," while the botanical name "*Trifolium*" refers to the three-lobed (trefoil) leaves. Red clover is extremely attractive to bumble bees, butterflies, and other beneficial insects; the honey from the flowers is extremely tasty. The dried flowers have a long history of use in Europe for wound healing and skin care. Red clover is now naturalized in North America and Australia and grown as a field crop.

252

SEE ALSO
Goldenseal, hyssop, echinacea, calendula, clary sage

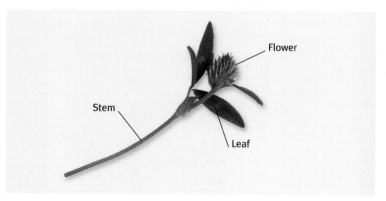

Flower

Stem

Leaf

RED CLOVER

Trifolium praetense

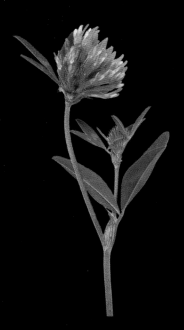

PART OF PLANT USED
Flowers

ACTIVE INGREDIENTS
Coumarins, flavonoids, glycosides, organic acids, pigment, tannins

COMMERCIALLY AVAILABLE AS
Dried herb, tablets, capsules, tincture

ACTIONS
Antispasmodic, astringent, expectorant, vulnerary

USED TO TREAT
Bronchitis, coughs, hoarseness of voice: an infusion of fresh or dried flowers with a teaspoon (5 ml) of honey soothes irritation and helps loosen catarrh.
Wounds, cuts: an infusion of fresh or dried flowers, cooled, makes an astringent and wound healing skin wash; a macerated oil with the flowers applied 2–3 times daily speeds healing (see page 298).
Eczema, psoriasis: a macerated oil made from fresh or dried flowers, as above, applied 2–3 times daily, helps heal deep cracks and areas of skin damage.
PMS/hormonal skin problems: tablets, capsules, or tincture taken as directed help heal hormonal skin blemishes and premenstrual imbalance.

CULINARY USE
None

SAFETY INFORMATION
No issues

TRIGONELLA FOENUM-GRAECUM
• FENUGREEK

This hardy annual herb grows up to 2 ft (60 cm) tall, with an erect, branching stem and leaves arranged in three lobes. It can be grown from seed in well-drained, nutrient-rich soil in full sun. It has pale yellow flowers with violet tips—these are unstalked, growing directly in the axils where the leaves and main stem meet. Curved pods containing aromatic seeds form later. The seeds—the main medicinal part—can then be collected and dried. The whole plant has a sharp aroma and makes an unusual addition to an herb garden.

The botanical name "*foenum-graecum*" literally means "Greek hay." This is said to reflect the ancient practice of mixing the plant with hay in horse fodder. "*Trigonella*" refers to the trifoliate arrangement of the leaves, resembling clover. Since ancient times, fenugreek seeds have been used throughout Europe, Asia, and the Far East, both in medicine and cooking. In traditional Chinese and Indian medicinal practice, they are used to cleanse the body and skin of impurities; they also have a reputed aphrodisiac effect.

SEE ALSO
Turmeric, cardamom, arnica, ginseng, saw palmetto

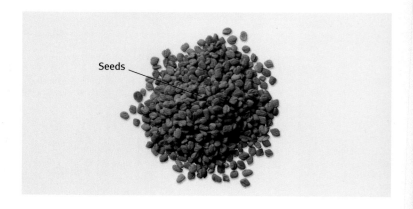

Seeds

FENUGREEK

Trigonella foenum-graecum

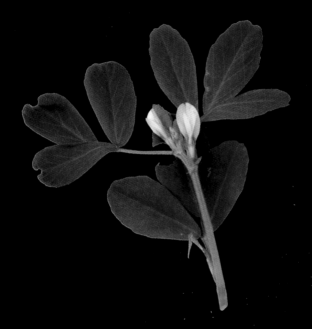

PART OF PLANT USED
Seeds

ACTIVE INGREDIENTS
Alkaloids, flavonoids, mucilage, steroidal saponins, vitamins A, B, and C

COMMERCIALLY AVAILABLE AS
Dried seeds, capsules, tablets

ACTIONS
Anti-inflammatory, digestive tonic, reproductive and sexual tonic

USED TO TREAT
Indigestion, Irritable Bowel Syndrome (IBS): capsules or tablets taken as directed are anti-inflammatory, easing pain and improving digestion.
Bruises, sprains or knocks: a macerated oil or ointment made with ground seeds (see pages 298–9) applied to injured areas reduces inflammation.
Impotence, male sexual dysfunction: traditional Chinese medicine regards fenugreek seeds as stimulants for male sexual energy; eating them or taking capsules can have a tonic effect.

CULINARY USE
Seeds can be sprouted and added to salads, while dried ground seeds add pungency to Indian curries, North African, and Middle Eastern dishes.

SAFETY INFORMATION
Fenugreek leaves or seeds should not be used medicinally during pregnancy because of potential hormonal effects. Culinary flavoring is safe.

TROPAEOLUM MAJUS
• NASTURTIUM

This lovely plant can grow as high as 10 ft (3 m), climbing on trailing stems. It has circular-shaped leaves with radiating veins, and brightly colored, orange or yellow flowers followed by round seeds. In northern latitudes it needs to be planted annually, although it will self-seed in hotter climates (originally native to South America, nasturtium was introduced to Spain from Peru in the 16th century). For medicinal purposes, obtain seeds of this species from a reputable supplier. Nasturtium is easy to grow from seed planted in late spring directly into the ground. It thrives in virtually any kind of soil in full sun or partial shade, although it needs watering regularly in hot weather. The edible flowers can be harvested as they come into bloom, as can the leaves, which are rich in vitamin C and iron. The seeds are useful medicinally, containing antiseptic ingredients.

The common name "nasturtium" comes from the Latin "*nasturcium*," which was given to various types of cress—this plant is closely related to watercress (*Nasturtium officinale*). After its arrival in Europe in the 16th century it soon naturalized itself and became a very popular garden plant, and by the 17th century it was appreciated as a salad ingredient, with pickled nasturtium seeds used as a seasoning similar to capers.

SEE ALSO
Tea tree, manuka, saw palmetto, goldenrod, parsley

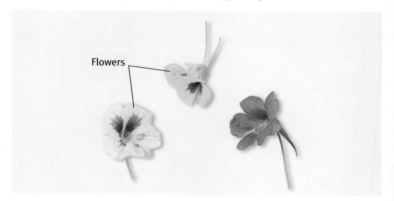

Flowers

NASTURTIUM

Tropaeolum majus

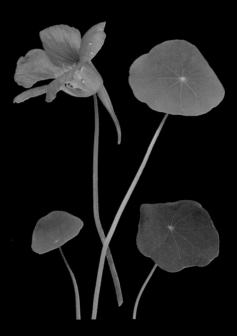

PART OF PLANT USED
Seeds

ACTIVE INGREDIENTS
Fatty oil, protein, volatile oil

COMMERCIALLY AVAILABLE AS
Not generally available commercially; best cultivated

ACTIONS
Powerful antiseptic, emollient

USED TO TREAT
Sore throats, bronchitis: an infusion of crushed seeds taken 2–3 times daily has a powerful effect on the bacteria that cause infections; also use as a gargle
Urinary-tract infections, prostatitis: an infusion of crushed seeds taken 2–3 times daily acts against urinary tract infections and clears them via the kidneys.

CULINARY USE
The fresh, green leaves add pungency to green salad combinations and the flowers are also edible, adding bright, contrasting color.

SAFETY INFORMATION
If you are on medication to treat urinary or prostate infections, only use nasturtium under professional supervision.

TURNERA DIFFUSA
• DAMIANA

This aromatic herb is native to Texas, Mexico, and Central America, thriving in a hot and humid environment. It grows up to 3 ft (1 m) tall, and its leaves are small and grouped in bunches, the undersides covered with silky hairs. The flowers are small and bright yellow, and they grow directly in the axils where the leaves and main stem meet. The seeds are small and curved. The whole plant is highly aromatic, smelling similar to camomile, indicating the presence of a volatile oil. With the intense interest in the commercial sale of the herb, distilled damiana essential oil is hard to obtain, because of the large quantities of plant material needed to yield useful amounts. The flowering tops of the plant, that is the stems, leaves, and blooms together, are harvested for medicinal purposes and mostly dried to make commercial herbal capsules and other preparations.

The native people of Central and South America have traditionally used damiana as a sexual tonic, leading to its reputation as an aphrodisiac. They brewed it as an infusion or smoked it like tobacco. Today it is mostly used as a nerve tonic to alleviate depression and states of anxiety.

SEE ALSO
Ginseng, saw palmetto, St. John's wort, hops, black cohosh

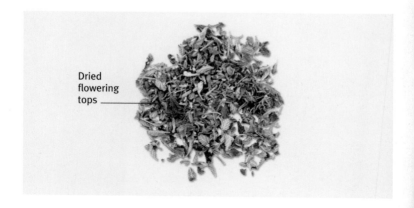

Dried
flowering
tops

DAMIANA

Turnera diffusa

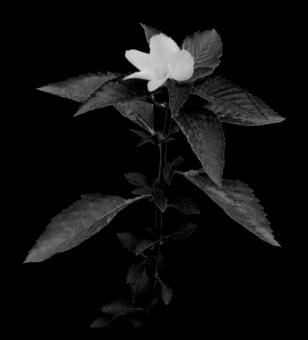

PART OF PLANT USED
Flowering tops

ACTIVE INGREDIENTS:
Glycoside, plant sterol, resin, volatile oil

COMMERCIALLY AVAILABLE AS
Tablets, capsules (occasionally as an essential oil)

ACTIONS
Anti-depressant, aphrodisiac, laxative, nerve tonic

USED TO TREAT
Anxiety, depression: tablets or capsules taken as directed ease mental stress and improve relaxation.
Impotence, frigidity, low libido: tablets or capsules taken as directed stimulate sexual energy and tone the reproductive system in both men and women.
Irregular menstruation: tablets or capsules taken as directed over at least three menstrual cycles help to balance the hormones and regulate menstrual rhythm.

CULINARY USE
None

SAFETY INFORMATION
Damiana may affect blood sugar levels, so it should be avoided by diabetics. Large doses can purge the bowels or cause headaches or insomnia. Best avoided in pregnancy because of the hormonal effects.

TUSSILAGO FARFARA
• COLTSFOOT

This tough, perennial herb often grows wild as a weed on bare waste ground, roadsides, and in woodland where the ground is very damp—it is found all over Europe and the British Isles. It grows from a large, branching root, with erect, purplish colored stems, culminating in yellow daisy-shaped flowers. Its large, fleshy, pale green leaves have darker, serrated edges; underneath they are white with a downy texture. The flower heads and young leaves were traditionally harvested in early spring to be used medicinally; the leaves are high in mucilage, which is a soothing ingredient that coats itself over enflamed tissues.

Colstfoot is an example of a medicinal plant that used to be highly regarded as an important respiratory remedy, as seen in the botanical name "*Tussilago*" from the Latin "*tussis*," meaning cough. The 17th-century English herbalist Nicholas Culpeper regarded it as a remedy for breathing difficulties such as asthma or wheezing. In more recent times, concerns have been raised about certain alkaloid compounds in the leaves that could cause liver damage, leading to the medicinal use and sale of the herb being banned in some countries. The hazards are still under dispute, but some medical herbalists still employ coltsfoot internally for short periods of time.

SEE ALSO
White horehound, pine, myrrh, Devil's claw, rosehip

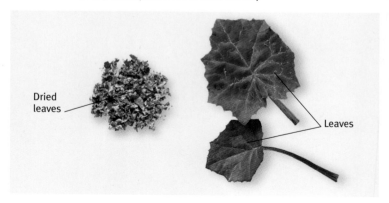

Dried leaves

Leaves

COLTSFOOT

Tussilago farfara

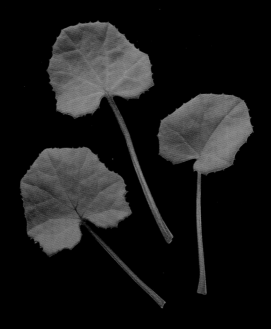

PART OF PLANT USED
Young leaves

ACTIVE INGREDIENTS
Bitters, alkaloids, mucilage, tannins, volatile oil

COMMERCIALLY AVAILABLE AS
Banned from sale in most countries

ACTIONS
Anti-inflammatory, astringent, expectorant

USED TO TREAT
Coughs, bronchitis, catarrh: syrup made from the young leaves may be taken under professional guidance for short periods to relieve chesty coughs.
Rheumatism, painful, swollen joints: infusion of the young leaves, cooled, can be applied to the joints as a compress to relieve painful swelling.

CULINARY USE
None

SAFETY INFORMATION
Coltsfoot is best employed by professional herbalists. Although it is easy to find growing wild, it is not recommended for self-administration. Because of the alkaloid content it should not be applied to open wounds.

ULMUS FULVA
• SLIPPERY ELM

Also known as Indian elm or moose elm, this is a tree native to many parts of North America. It grows up to 60 ft (18 m) tall with very rough bark on its trunk and branches. The buds are covered with dense, yellow fibers, and the leaves are long with toothed edges, and hairy on both sides. The most important part of the slippery elm is its inner bark, which is collected in spring from the larger branches and trunk; it is tough yet flexible, with a reddish brown color. It smells similar to fenugreek (see pages 254–5) and has a very bland taste. The bark is dried and ground—coarse grade is used to make medicinal poultices and fine grade is used to make herbal supplements or a drink.

Dried and ground slippery elm bark is a valuable food and medicine—the inner bark is a source of very soothing mucilage that calms inflammation. It is also very nutritious in similar ways to oatmeal—it can be eaten as a kind of porridge as well as taken as a remedy. It helps to counteract inflammation inside the digestive tract and is very valuable as a supportive remedy in convalescence, when eating and assimilation may be difficult—the mucilage in slippery elm helps food to travel through the digestive tract.

SEE ALSO

Aloe vera, oat, fenugreek, echinacea, German camomile

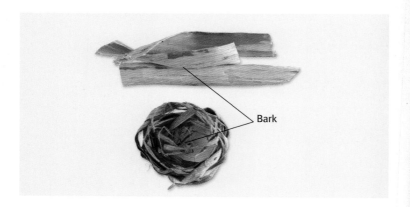

Bark

262

SLIPPERY ELM

Ulmus fulva

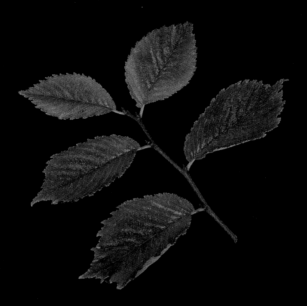

PART OF PLANT USED
Inner bark

ACTIVE INGREDIENTS
Mucilage, starch, tannin

COMMERCIALLY AVAILABLE AS
Capsules, powder, drink

ACTIONS
Anti-inflammatory, soothing, mucilaginous

USED TO TREAT
Colic, colitis, Irritable Bowel Syndrome (IBS): capsules taken as directed, or slippery elm drink taken 2–3 times daily soothes the lining of the digestive tract.
Convalescence: thin porridge (see below) taken 2–3 times daily strengthens the digestive tract and assists recovery.
Boils, infected wounds, splinters: ointment of slippery elm applied 2–3 times daily to affected areas draws out infection or foreign objects.
Wounds, burns: a slippery elm poultice draws out infection and soothes inflammation.

CULINARY USE
The powder can be mixed into a thin porridge with added nutmeg or cinnamon to make an easily digestible food.

SAFETY INFORMATION
No issues

URTICA DIOTICA
• NETTLE

This vigorous plant is unlikely to be cultivated in a garden as it spreads very efficiently on long creeping roots and can be invasive. Its stems can grow to 5 ft (1.5 m) tall. The dull green leaves have toothed edges and are covered in stinging hairs, and in late summer small, yellowish flowers appear. Nettles prefer moist soil, in sun or shade. If you have a lot of them you can make a nitrogen-rich plant food—half fill a bucket with leaves, then fill it completely with water and leave outside for a week, to produce a wonderfully pungent green liquid. Young, spring nettle stems are used for culinary purposes and medicinally. The smaller species, *Urtica urens*, is used to prepare the homeopathic remedy "urtica."

For hundreds of years nettles have been regarded as a valuable medicine to treat lung complaints and also to get rid of poison in the system. The name "nettle" is from the Anglo-Saxon word for the plant, "*netele*," which is related to the word for needle—nettle stems yield long fibers which were once used for sewing or making sacking.

SEE ALSO

Yarrow, burdock, horsetail, agnus castus, Roman camomile

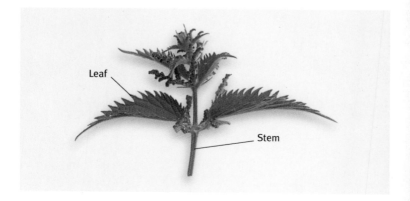

Leaf

Stem

NETTLE

Urtica diotica

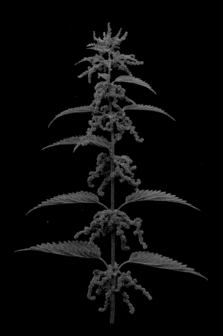

PART OF PLANT USED
Young leaves

ACTIVE INGREDIENTS
Formic acid, histamine, minerals
(especially iron and sulfur), tannins,
vitamins

COMMERCIALLY AVAILABLE AS
Dried herb, tea, tablets, tincture

ACTIONS
Astringent, antirheumatic, blood
purifying

USED TO TREAT
Gout, rheumatism, arthritis: tablets, capsules or tincture help to relieve the pain
of rheumatic conditions and stimulate
the circulation.

Anemia: the mineral content of nettle
makes it a good tonic to the blood; take
capsules, tablets, or tincture as directed,
or eat young leaves (see below).
*Excess menstrual bleeding, irregular
periods:* tablets, capsules, or tincture
taken regularly over a minimum of
three cycles can help regulate excess or
irregular bleeding.
Dandruff, scaling scalp: an infusion of
young leaves can be poured over the
hair and rubbed into the scalp to help
ease irritation.

CULINARY USE
Young nettle leaves can be boiled and
served like spinach or made into a soup.

SAFETY INFORMATION
No issues

VACCINIUM MACROCARPON
• CRANBERRY

Cranberry shrubs are low-growing, up to a height of 8 in (20 cm), with a creeping habit rather like vines. They thrive in acidic bogs in cooler locations throughout the northern hemisphere. Though some species are found in Europe, this one is native to North America and parts of Canada. The shrub produces slender, wiry stems and small, evergreen leaves. The flowers are dark pink in color, becoming a large berry that is initially white and then turns red as it ripens. Cranberries are an important commercial crop in areas of the United States, such as New Jersey, Minnesota, Washington, and Wisconsin. The berries are processed and made into juice, cranberry sauce, and dried cranberries, sweetened with sugar.

For centuries, cranberries have been collected and eaten by native peoples in northern countries such as Russia, as well as parts of North America and the Arctic, as a valuable source of vitamin C. Medicinally, the berries are of interest because they help to reduce urinary-tract infections. In recent years commercial interest has risen in the fatty oil contained in cranberry seeds; this contains a good balance of the fatty acids Omega 3, 6, and 9.

SEE ALSO

Bearberry/uva ursi, parsley, pau d'arco, echinacea, rosehip

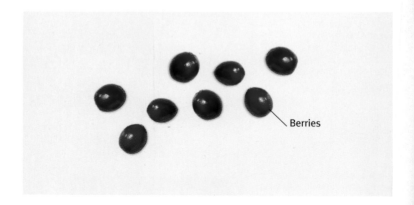

Berries

CRANBERRY

Vaccinium macrocarpon

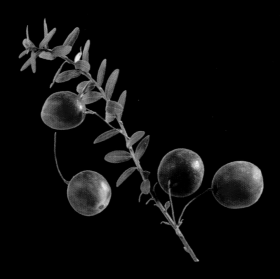

PARTS OF PLANT USED
Berries, seeds

ACTIVE INGREDIENTS
Berries—carotenoids, vitamin C;
seeds—Omega 3, 6, and 9 fatty acids

COMMERCIALLY AVAILABLE AS
Fresh or dried berries, tablets, capsules,
juice, oil capsules

ACTIONS
Berries—antiseptic, antioxidant,
diuretic; seeds—anti-inflammatory,
nerve tonic

USED TO TREAT
Urinary tract infections: juice taken twice
daily, or capsules or tablets as directed
help to cleanse the urinary tract.

Low immunity: juice taken twice daily
is a valuable source of vitamin C.
Inflammatory arthritis/swollen joints:
cranberry seed oil is reputed to have an
anti-inflammatory effect thanks to the
Omega fatty acids it contains.

CULINARY USE
Fresh berries can be made into jelly,
sauce, or relish.

SAFETY INFORMATION
Because of cranberries' anticoagulant
properties, drinking the juice or
taking the berries medicinally is
not recommended for people on
anticoagulant drugs.

VALERIANA OFFICINALIS
• VALERIAN

This tall, hardy, perennial herb grows up to 5 ft (1.5 m) tall. Its extensive root system produces angular, erect, furrowed stems. The leaves have between seven and thirteen leaflets, and the small flowers are pinkish white and densely packed. A red, ornamental valerian exists called *Centranthus ruber*, although it has no medicinal value — *Valeriana officinalis* is the healing plant. Valerian grows wild in damp meadows and ditches or near streams. In the garden it needs fertile, moist soil and full sun. It can be sown from seed in spring or existing plants can be dug up in fall, the roots separated into two or three clumps and replanted. Once established it can be invasive. Roots need to be at least two years old for medicinal use and need to be dried before making preparations.

In ancient Greece valerian was known as "*phu,*" perhaps because of its strong odor. However, by medieval times, it had acquired the common name "all heal," and was particularly valued for its sedative effects on the nervous system. The name "*Valeriana*" is possibly derived from the Latin "*valere*," meaning "to be healthy." Today valerian is used in many herbal tea and tablet combinations as a natural aid for sleeping problems, mental stress, and tension.

SEE ALSO

Oat, hops, melissa, St. John's wort, lavender

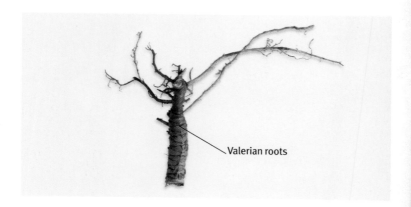

Valerian roots

VALERIAN

Valeriana officinalis

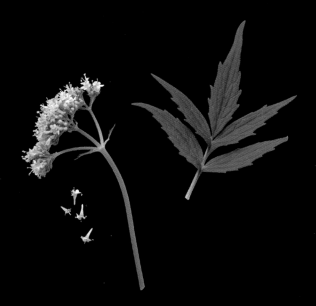

PART OF PLANT USED
Roots

ACTIVE INGREDIENTS
Alkaloids, bitters, tannins, volatile oil

COMMERCIALLY AVAILABLE AS
Dried root, tea, capsules, tincture

ACTIONS
Antispasmodic, sedative

USED TO TREAT
Insomnia: capsules, tablets, or tincture taken as directed can increase relaxation and help sleeping problems (see safety information).
Nervous stress, tension: capsules, tablets, or tincture taken as directed can help to ease anxiety and mental pressure (see safety information).
Headaches, migraine: capsules, tablets, or tincture taken as directed can ease spasmodic pain and improve general relaxation (see safety note below).

CULINARY USE
None

SAFETY INFORMATION
Do not use alongside conventional pain-killing drugs. If you are on medication for migraine or insomnia take medical advice before using valerian. Long-term use of the herb is not advised—if your condition does not improve then consult a professional herbalist for guidance.

VERBASCUM THAPSUS
• MULLEIN

This plant belongs to a vast family of *Verbascums*, with more than 200 species; these plants are found all over Europe, Asia, and North Africa. *Verbascum thapsus* or "great mullein" is found in temperate latitudes across North America, Europe, and as far afield as the Himalayas. In its first year of growth it only produces a rosette of leaves that are at least 6 in (15 cm) long, thick-textured, and covered with white hairs on both sides. The following spring a stout, hairy stem rises from the middle of the rosette of leaves, with smaller, alternate, hairy leaves. At the top of the stalk, which can reach up to 4 ft (1.2 m) in height, a thickly crowded flower spike forms, covered in bright yellow flowers. The leaves and flowers are both useful medicinally—mullein is very mucilaginous, making it a soothing remedy for coughs and respiratory problems.

In the past, dried mullein was valued as tinder for starting fires, because its hairs would catch light very easily. This led to it being given the common name, the "candlewick plant." It was regularly fed to cattle to protect them from diseases of the lungs. In the 19th century it gained popularity as a garden plant specifically being used to make cough syrup to help diseases of the lungs, such as consumption.

SEE ALSO
White horehound, nasturtium, goldenseal, olive, oak bark

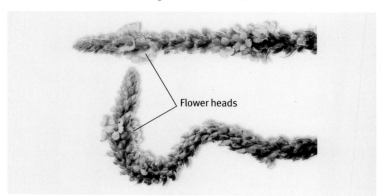

Flower heads

MULLEIN
Verbascum thapsus

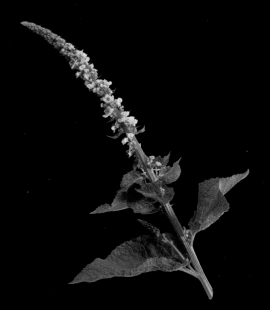

PART OF PLANT USED
Leaves, flowers

ACTIVE INGREDIENTS
Leaves—bitters, mucilage, tannins; flowers—gum, pigment, minerals, resin, volatile oil

COMMERCIALLY AVAILABLE AS
Dried herb, tablets, macerated oil, cough medicine

ACTIONS
Diuretic, expectorant, mucilaginous

USED TO TREAT
Coughs, bronchitis, catarrh: cough medicine or tablets taken as directed help coat the respiratory-tract lining, soothing coughs and expelling mucus.

Earache: macerated oil (see page 298) of mullein can be dropped into the ear 2–3 times daily to reduce inflammation and heal minor infections.
Boils, skin sores, chilblains: macerated mullein oil applied 2–3 times daily eases pain and heals infection.

CULINARY USE
None

SAFETY INFORMATION
Some species of *Verbascum* look similar to this one and are poisonous; picking in the wild is not advised.

VERBENA OFFICINALIS
• VERVAIN

This perennial herb grows up to 2 ft (60 cm) tall with tough, four-sided, erect stems. The foliage is sparse, made up of long, oval leaves with toothed but rounded edges, arranged in pairs. The flowers are small and pink or lilac in color. The whole plant is covered with light, silky hairs. Vervain is native to southern Europe and was probably introduced to Britain by the Romans (it can be found wild in southern England and parts of Wales). It thrives in sheltered spots out of the wind, and prefers well-drained soil. Vervain's flowering tops are the medicinally active part and are collected just as the flowers come into bloom.

Vervain was a very important herb in Roman spiritual practice, used to decorate altars in temples and make floral wreaths for important feasts. In medieval times it was considered an important ingredient in love potions, and it features frequently in ancient texts relating to witchcraft and magic. It was believed to offer protection against evil spirits, spells, and even the plague. Today it is mostly used in herbal medicine to help conditions of the nervous system, and support liver function.

SEE ALSO
Yellow gentian, fennel, slippery elm, oat, feverfew

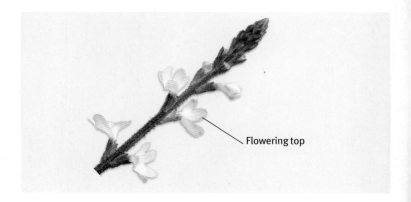

Flowering top

VERVAIN

Verbena officinalis

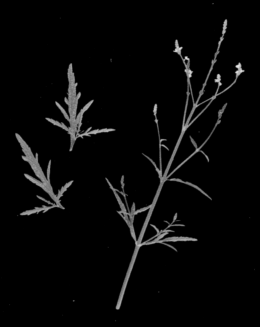

PART OF PLANT USED
Flowering tops

ACTIVE INGREDIENTS
Glycosides, minerals, mucilage, saponins, tannins, volatile oil

COMMERCIALLY AVAILABLE AS
Dried herb, tablets, tincture

ACTIONS
Antispasmodic, astringent, digestive tonic, diuretic, sedative, uterine tonic

USED TO TREAT
Sluggish digestion, poor liver function: tablets or tincture taken as directed stimulate liver function and improve digestive processes.
Convalescence, low physical energy: tablets or tincture taken as directed help support the digestion if it is weakened after illness.
Insomnia, nervous stress, and tension: tablets or tincture taken as directed ease mental stress and improve relaxation.
Headaches, migraine: tablets or tincture taken as directed have a sedative and antispasmodic effect, increasing relaxation and easing pain.

CULINARY USE
None

SAFETY INFORMATION
Avoid during pregnancy. However, it can be taken in labor to help stimulate contractions (seek professional guidance from an herbalist).

VIOLA ODORATA
• WILD VIOLET

This perennial herb grows up to 4 in (10 cm) tall. It has short, thick roots and spreads by sending out feelers called "runners" that root again at the tips, making new plants. The leaves are soft, toothed, and rounded, and the flowering stalks rise out of the center of a rosette of leaves. The tiny, deep purple blooms have a delicate aroma. Violets are a spring flower, growing in many parts of the world including Europe, the United States, Asia, and China. The plants form carpets of purple blooms, typically in damp, shady conditions. They can be cultivated in cool, dark spots in a garden. There are hundreds of ornamental varieties of *Viola*—make sure seeds are this species if you want plants for medicinal use. The leaves and scented flowers have medicinal properties—currently the plant is commercially cultivated in southern France for herbal and perfumery use.

The ancient Greeks regarded violets as a tonic for the heart, to soothe deep emotions such as grief, or to calm anger. The plant has an overall cooling effect on body and mind. In traditional Chinese medicine, leaves and roots are used to take the heat and swelling out of knocks and injuries. Soaking violet flowers in milk was a popular skin and beauty treatment in the early Middle Ages.

SEE ALSO

Goldenseal, cornflower, echinacea, Roman camomile, arnica

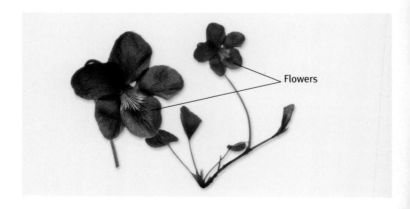

Flowers

WILD VIOLET
Viola odorata

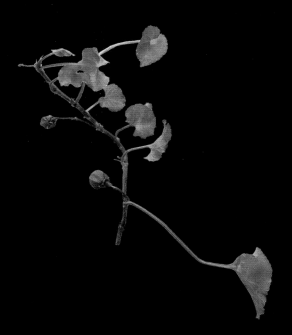

PART OF PLANT USED
Flowers, leaves

ACTIVE INGREDIENTS
Glycoside, mucilage, pigments, saponins

COMMERCIALLY AVAILABLE AS
Tea, face cream, absolute (perfume extract from the flowers, using solvent), cough syrup

ACTIONS
Cooling, expectorant, diuretic

USED TO TREAT
Sore throats, mouth ulcers: syrup of the leaves and flowers taken 2–3 times daily soothes irritated membranes at the back of the throat.
Coughs, bronchitis: syrup taken 2–3 times daily soothes spasmodic coughing and helps expel mucus.
Colds, fevers: an infusion of leaves and flowers, cooled, can be used as a cold compress to reduce fever.
Swelling, sprains, injuries: an infusion of the leaves, cooled, can be used as a compress to reduce swelling and heat.

CULINARY USE
Flowers can be candied as cake decorations.

SAFETY INFORMATION
Violet root is a strong purgative and should only be used under professional guidance.

VITEX AGNUS CASTUS
• AGNUS CASTUS

This fragrant, deciduous shrub grows to heights of 3–12 ft (1–4 m) depending on its environment—in a garden it will grow taller, in a rocky environment it may adopt a more creeping habit. It is native to southern Europe, western Asia, and North America. Its young twigs are grayish, with sharply toothed, lance-shaped leaves, dark green above and gray below. It produces clusters of bluish-pink, scented blooms that become small, dark, purple, aromatic berries. It likes a dry and sunny location, and does well in coastal environments, even in poor soil. The berries are the medicinal part of the plant and are collected at the end of the flowering season.

The Latin name of the plant, *agnus castus*, means "chaste lamb," and "*Vitex*" could be linked to the verb "*vito*" meaning "I avoid," possibly alluding to a long-standing belief that the bush had an anaphrodisiac effect—one of its common names is "chasteberry." Modern research has identified a hormone-regulating effect from the berries, making them helpful to deal with female reproductive problems such as irregular menstruation or excess bleeding. Today agnus castus is commonly used as a natural support for women going through the menopause.

SEE ALSO
Black cohosh, wild yam, rose, sage, fennel

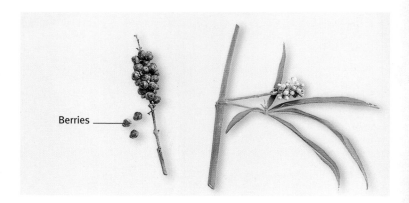

Berries

AGNUS CASTUS

Vitex agnus castus

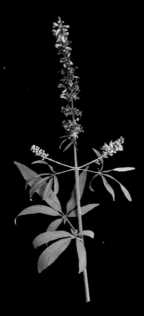

PART OF PLANT USED
Berries

ACTIVE INGREDIENTS
Bitters, glycosides, flavonoids, volatile oil

COMMERCIALLY AVAILABLE AS
Tablets, tincture

ACTIONS
Hormonal regulator, galactogogue

USED TO TREAT
Irregular or heavy periods: tablets or tincture taken as directed can balance hormone levels, helping to regulate cycles and levels of bleeding; it is slow acting and needs to be taken regularly for several months.

Menopausal symptoms: tablets or capsules taken as directed help maintain hormone balance and ease problems such as low energy and mood swings.
Lack of breast milk: agnus castus has been shown to increase levels of prolactin, the hormone that governs the release of breast milk. However, professional advice on dosage should be sought when breast-feeding.

CULINARY USE
None

SAFETY INFORMATION
Use of agnus castus is not advised during pregnancy because of its hormone-regulating influence. Avoid if you are taking hormone replacement therapy (HRT) or the contraceptive pill.

VITIS VINIFERA
• GRAPESEED

This is a vigorous climbing plant, capable of spreading itself over an area covering 30 ft (10 m) square if left unpruned. It produces very large leaves with toothed edges, and its woody stems can easily expand to 3 ft (1 m) in diameter. Spikes of tiny, yellow flowers appear in late spring, becoming tiny, unripe, green fruit that swell over the summer to ripen in September and early fall. Originally native to southern European countries such as Greece, as well as parts of North Africa, grapevines have been transplanted and successfully naturalized into northern Europe, Australia, and North and South America during the growth of the worldwide winemaking industry. Grape seeds contain a fatty oil and antioxidant compounds, which help to detoxify the body and tone the circulation. They are processed as a by-product after grape harvesting and pressing.

The grapevine is one of the most significant plants in human history—it has been cultivated since antiquity for its fruit and for winemaking. Ripe grapes, an excellent source of vitamin C, also have a gently diuretic effect on the system and are excellent in convalescence. Grapeseed extract is becoming popular as a dietary supplement because of its antioxidant properties; it is also rich in polyphenols that strengthen the heart and circulation, and tone the veins.

SEE ALSO
Horse chestnut, hawthorn, myrrh, cayenne pepper, pine

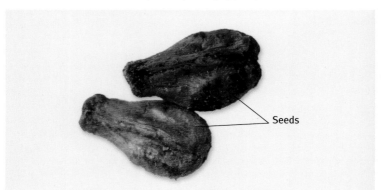

Seeds

GRAPESEED
Vitis vinifera

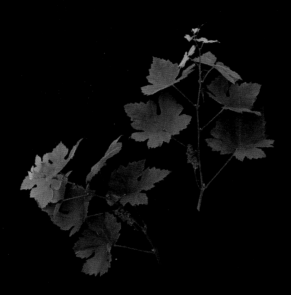

PART OF PLANT USED
Seeds

ACTIVE INGREDIENTS
Polyphenols, fatty oil rich in linoleic acid

COMMERCIALLY AVAILABLE AS
Capsules, liquid oil

ACTIONS
Anticoagulant, antioxidant, vein tonic

USED TO TREAT
Broken veins, varicose veins: capsules taken as directed help to strengthen and tone the walls of the veins, limiting damage.
Poor circulation: capsules taken as directed tone and strengthen the heart and circulation.

Toxic build-up from pollution, drugs, tobacco: the antioxidant properties of grapeseed capsules, taken as directed, help minimize internal damage at the cellular level.

CULINARY USE
Grapeseed oil is light textured and can be used in cooking or salad dressings.

SAFETY INFORMATION
Because of the anticoagulant effect, grapeseed extract is not recommended for people on anticoagulant drugs such as Warfarin; if in any doubt please seek professional medical advice.

ZINGIBER OFFICINALE
• GINGER

This perennial plant has a very fleshy, pungent, and juicy root (rhizome), which is dug up and used fresh in cooking or dried for use as a spice or in medicines. It produces long, elegant pairs of lance-shaped leaves on stems up to 4 ft (1.2 m) tall, and very aromatic flowers on cones separate to the leaves. It requires fertile, very rich, moist soil and a humid tropical climate. It can be grown in a greenhouse or conservatory, but regular spraying with water is needed to stop the leaves from drying out.

Ginger root has been used for millennia in tropical Asia, China, and India as an aphrodisiac and a vital culinary spice, as well as an important medicinal remedy for diarrhea, malaria, colds, and stomach disorders. In Europe ginger is mentioned in medicinal texts from Anglo-Saxon times (10th century CE), and it was probably brought west along early trade routes. Ginger has been a popular ingredient in sweet and savory cooking from medieval times onwards. In the 16th century the Spaniards transported ginger to the West Indies and the Americas for cultivation, where it now flourishes.

SEE ALSO
Cardamom, turmeric, peppermint, myrtle, rosemary

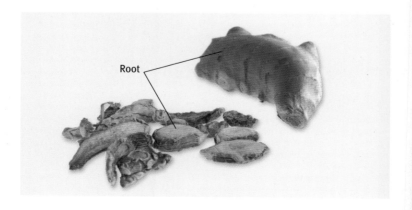

Root

GINGER

Zingiber officinale

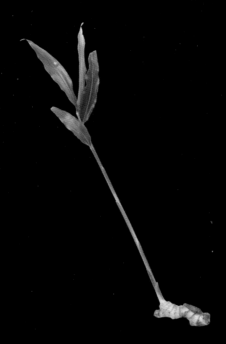

PART OF PLANT USED
Root

ACTIVE INGREDIENTS
Amino acids, resin, starch, vitamins, volatile oil

COMMERCIALLY AVAILABLE AS
Fresh and dried root, crystallized ginger, essential oil, ground spice, tea, capsules, tablets

ACTIONS
Circulation stimulant, diaphoretic, digestive tonic

USED TO TREAT
Indigestion, nausea, travel sickness, morning sickness: tablets taken as directed or tea made with 1 teaspoon (5 g) of fresh, chopped, root ginger and a teaspoon of honey can be drunk 2–3 times daily to ease nausea and indigestion symptoms.
Influenza, colds, coughs: ginger tea (as above) taken 2–3 times daily promotes sweating and helps the body through viral episodes, as well as easing coughs.
Muscular aches and pains: 2 drops of essential oil in 1 teaspoon (5 ml) of sunflower oil massaged into affected areas eases pain.

CULINARY USE
Dried ginger adds a spicy note to biscuits and cakes; fresh, chopped, root ginger is an essential flavoring in Asian cooking.

SAFETY INFORMATION
No issues

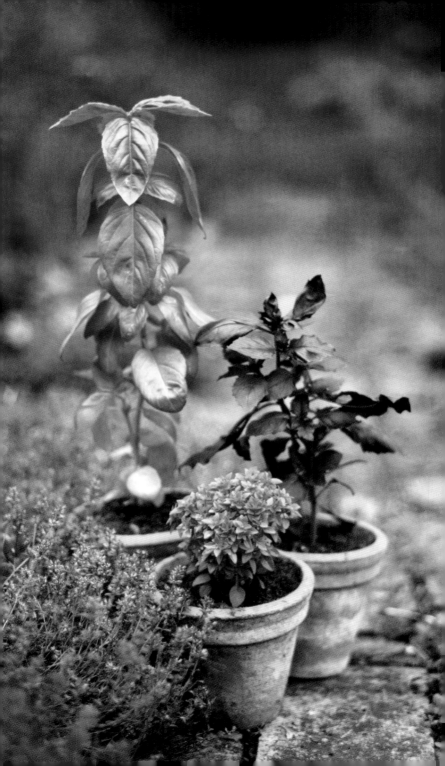

THE HERB GALLERY

On the following pages, all 130 herbs featured in the Directory are presented in miniature, listed alphabetically by Latin name, demonstrating the huge diversity and beauty of herbs.

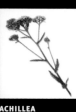

ACHILLEA MILLEFOLIUM
YARROW

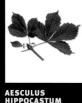

AESCULUS HIPPOCASTUM
HORSE CHESTNUT

ALCHEMILLA VULGARIS
LADY'S MANTLE

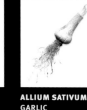

ALLIUM SATIVUM
GARLIC

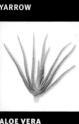

ALOE VERA
ALOE VERA

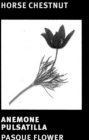

ANEMONE PULSATILLA
PASQUE FLOWER

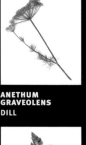

ANETHUM GRAVEOLENS
DILL

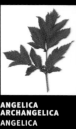

ANGELICA ARCHANGELICA
ANGELICA

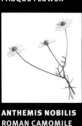

ANGELICA SINENSIS
DONG QUAI

ANTHEMIS NOBILIS
ROMAN CAMOMILE

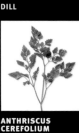

ANTHRISCUS CEREFOLIUM

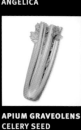

APIUM GRAVEOLENS
CELERY SEED

**ARTEMISIA
DRACUNCULUS**
TARRAGON

AVENA SATIVA
OAT

BELLIS PERENNIS
DAISY

BETULA PENDULA
SILVER BIRCH

**BORAGO
OFFICINALIS**
BORAGE

BRASSICA NIGRA
MUSTARD SEED
(BLACK)

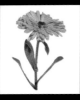

**CALENDULA
OFFICINALIS**
CALENDULA

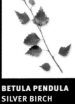

**CAPSICUM
FRUTESCENS**
CAYENNE PEPPER

**CASSIA
ANGUSTIFOLIA**
SENNA

CENTAUREA CYANUS
CORNFLOWER

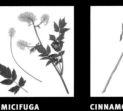

**CIMICIFUGA
RACEMOSA**
BLACK COHOSH

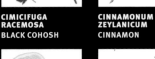

**CINNAMONUM
ZEYLANICUM**
CINNAMON

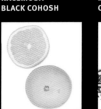

CITRUS AURANTIUM

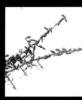

CITRUS LIMONUM

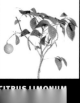

CITRUS X PARADISI

COMMIPHORA

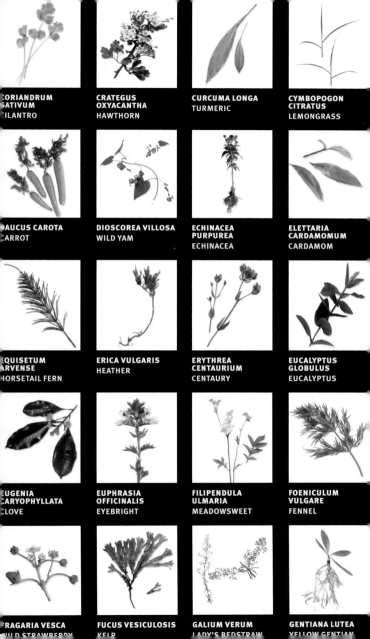

CORIANDRUM SATIVUM
CILANTRO

CRATEGUS OXYACANTHA
HAWTHORN

CURCUMA LONGA
TURMERIC

CYMBOPOGON CITRATUS
LEMONGRASS

DAUCUS CAROTA
CARROT

DIOSCOREA VILLOSA
WILD YAM

ECHINACEA PURPUREA
ECHINACEA

ELETTARIA CARDAMOMUM
CARDAMOM

EQUISETUM ARVENSE
HORSETAIL FERN

ERICA VULGARIS
HEATHER

ERYTHREA CENTAURIUM
CENTAURY

EUCALYPTUS GLOBULUS
EUCALYPTUS

EUGENIA CARYOPHYLLATA
CLOVE

EUPHRASIA OFFICINALIS
EYEBRIGHT

FILIPENDULA ULMARIA
MEADOWSWEET

FOENICULUM VULGARE
FENNEL

FRAGARIA VESCA
WILD STRAWBERRY

FUCUS VESICULOSIS
KELP

GALIUM VERUM
LADY'S BEDSTRAW

GENTIANA LUTEA
YELLOW GENTIAN

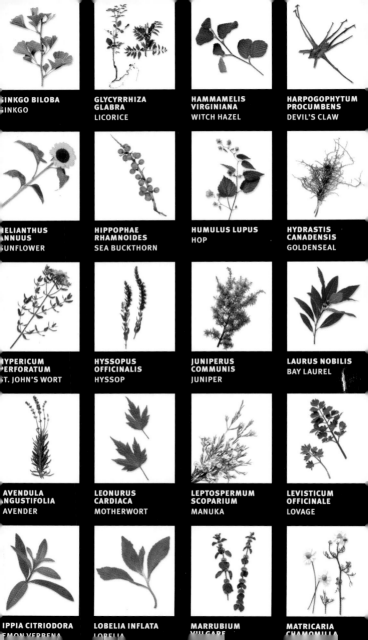

GINKGO BILOBA
GINKGO

GLYCYRRHIZA GLABRA
LICORICE

HAMMAMELIS VIRGINIANA
WITCH HAZEL

HARPOGOPHYTUM PROCUMBENS
DEVIL'S CLAW

HELIANTHUS ANNUUS
SUNFLOWER

HIPPOPHAE RHAMNOIDES
SEA BUCKTHORN

HUMULUS LUPUS
HOP

HYDRASTIS CANADENSIS
GOLDENSEAL

HYPERICUM PERFORATUM
ST. JOHN'S WORT

HYSSOPUS OFFICINALIS
HYSSOP

JUNIPERUS COMMUNIS
JUNIPER

LAURUS NOBILIS
BAY LAUREL

LAVENDULA ANGUSTIFOLIA
LAVENDER

LEONURUS CARDIACA
MOTHERWORT

LEPTOSPERMUM SCOPARIUM
MANUKA

LEVISTICUM OFFICINALE
LOVAGE

LIPPIA CITRIODORA
LEMON VERBENA

LOBELIA INFLATA
LOBELIA

MARRUBIUM VULGARE

MATRICARIA CHAMOMILLA

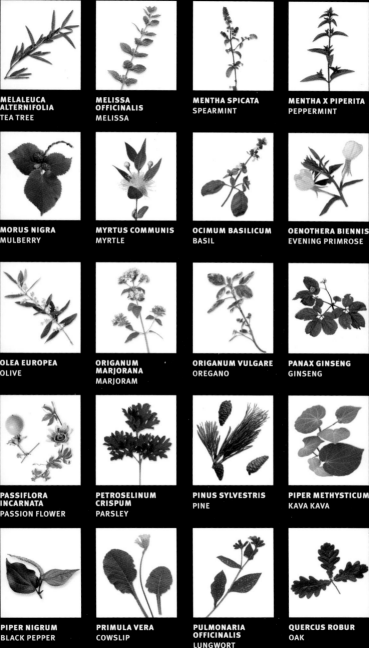

MELALEUCA ALTERNIFOLIA
TEA TREE

MELISSA OFFICINALIS
MELISSA

MENTHA SPICATA
SPEARMINT

MENTHA X PIPERITA
PEPPERMINT

MORUS NIGRA
MULBERRY

MYRTUS COMMUNIS
MYRTLE

OCIMUM BASILICUM
BASIL

OENOTHERA BIENNIS
EVENING PRIMROSE

OLEA EUROPEA
OLIVE

ORIGANUM MARJORANA
MARJORAM

ORIGANUM VULGARE
OREGANO

PANAX GINSENG
GINSENG

PASSIFLORA INCARNATA
PASSION FLOWER

PETROSELINUM CRISPUM
PARSLEY

PINUS SYLVESTRIS
PINE

PIPER METHYSTICUM
KAVA KAVA

PIPER NIGRUM
BLACK PEPPER

PRIMULA VERA
COWSLIP

PULMONARIA OFFICINALIS
LUNGWORT

QUERCUS ROBUR
OAK

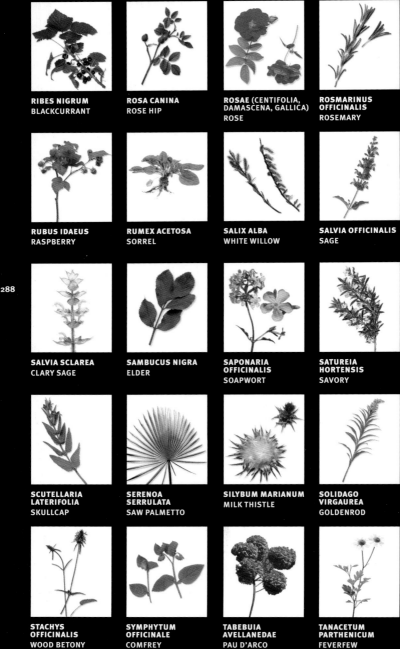

RIBES NIGRUM
BLACKCURRANT

ROSA CANINA
ROSE HIP

ROSAE (CENTIFOLIA, DAMASCENA, GALLICA)
ROSE

ROSMARINUS OFFICINALIS
ROSEMARY

RUBUS IDAEUS
RASPBERRY

RUMEX ACETOSA
SORREL

SALIX ALBA
WHITE WILLOW

SALVIA OFFICINALIS
SAGE

SALVIA SCLAREA
CLARY SAGE

SAMBUCUS NIGRA
ELDER

SAPONARIA OFFICINALIS
SOAPWORT

SATUREIA HORTENSIS
SAVORY

SCUTELLARIA LATERIFOLIA
SKULLCAP

SERENOA SERRULATA
SAW PALMETTO

SILYBUM MARIANUM
MILK THISTLE

SOLIDAGO VIRGAUREA
GOLDENROD

STACHYS OFFICINALIS
WOOD BETONY

SYMPHYTUM OFFICINALE
COMFREY

TABEBUIA AVELLANEDAE
PAU D'ARCO

TANACETUM PARTHENICUM
FEVERFEW

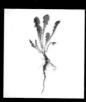

TARAXACUM OFFICINALE
DANDELION

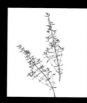

THYMUS VULGARIS
THYME

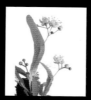

TILIA CORDATA
LIME FLOWER

TRIFOLIUM PRAETENSE
RED CLOVER

TRIGONELLA FOENUM-GRAECUM
FENUGREEK

TROPAEOLUM MAJUS
NASTURTIUM

TURNERA DIFFUSA
DAMIANA

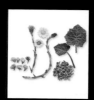

TUSSILAGO FARFARA
COLTSFOOT

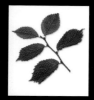

ULMUS FULVA
SLIPPERY ELM

URTICA DIOTICA
NETTLE

VACCINIUM MACROCARPON
CRANBERRY

VALERIANA OFFICINALIS
VALERIAN

289

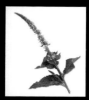

VERBASCUM THAPSUS
MULLEIN

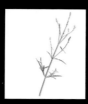

VERBENA OFFICINALIS
VERVAIN

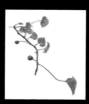

VIOLA ODORATA
WILD VIOLET

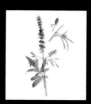

VITEX AGNUS CASTUS
AGNUS CASTUS

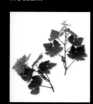

VITIS VINIFERA
GRAPESEED

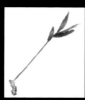

ZINGIBER OFFICINALE
GINGER

CONTAINER HERB GARDENING

A collection of herbs in different-sized pots creates an attractive display in a small space. If you don't have a garden, then growing herbs in pots is a simple and easy way to enjoy fresh herbs all year round.

CHOOSE YOUR CONTAINER

Many herbs have compact, attractive shapes, so they do well in pots and containers. Terracotta pots are best for herbs because they are porous—most herbs do not like to be too moist, and plastic pots retain water. Make sure you plant your herbs in pots large enough for their roots to spread well, particularly if you want them to grow for a few years.

CHOICES OF HERBS

It is best to stick to one herb per pot, although, for a change, you could try planting several species of basil (*Ocimum basilicum*) in the same pot—such as "Purple Ruffles" with a spicy aroma, or "Genovese" which is highly fragrant, or the little Greek basil "Minimum."

PREPARING AND MAINTAINING POTS

Put a layer of rough stones in the base of the pot for good drainage and air circulation. Fill the pot with a balanced mixture ideal for herb growth—one third topsoil, one third compost, and one third coarse sand. Herbs in pots use up nutrients quickly, so you need to give them liquid feed every six weeks or so in the growing season. In the heat of summer, water your pots, but not too much, just enough to keep the surface moist.

LEFT: Herbs thrive in pots and containers. Being porous, terracotta pots work best, allowing the herbs to drain

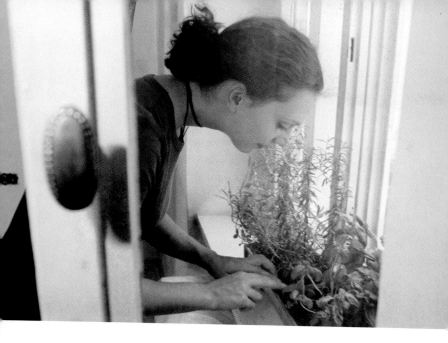

CHOOSE YOUR SPACE

ABOVE: A windowsill makes an excellent location for an herb container—choose a south facing, sunny ledge

Container herb gardens can be created in very small spaces. Mediterranean herbs in particular love to be in the sun as much as possible, and add their wonderful aromas and attractive appearance to sheltered areas.

Windowsills: use sunny, south-facing ledges to arrange pots of herbs such as thyme, sage, or sweet marjoram to be cut fresh for cooking. Chives work well in a pot, as do tarragon and cilantro. Arrange your herbs close to your kitchen for ease of access.

Courtyards: in southern Europe, stone-walled courtyards act like sun traps and are often homes for an array of pots and climbing plants such as passion flower, a varied collection of aromatic shrubs like myrtle or bay for large tubs, or large pots of rosemary, basil, and fennel for kitchen and medicinal use.

Balconies: these work very well as herb-growing spaces, particularly if the sun reaches them for at least part of the day. Fixing a trellis to a side wall would allow a vine to be planted in a pot for a lovely foliage display and edible fruit.

Front porches: sheltered porches can make excellent protective spaces for tender plants, almost like mini-conservatories. Aromatic, fragrant herbs such as lavender, scented geraniums, or bay trees are very attractive outside your front door, and all of these work well in pots or tubs.

CREATING YOUR OWN HERB GARDEN

It pays to think about what kind of herbs you want to grow and how you want to use them. Consider how much space you have and how you will lay out your herbs. Designing an herb garden is a lovely, creative task.

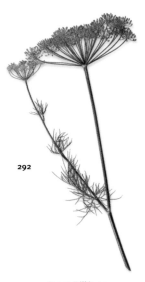

ABOVE: Dill is an excellent choice to plant in full sun

PLANNING AN HERB GARDEN

Creating a useful garden that is relevant to you means you will be out in it all the time and interacting with your plants regularly.

- If you want to use fresh herbs in cooking, and also to dry or preserve some for the winter months, consider herbs such as rosemary, basil, thyme, tarragon, fennel, marjoram, sage, and garlic.
- If you want to grow herbs to use for general health, to make teas and other preparations, then consider German camomile, feverfew, Lady's mantle, Roman camomile, and echinacea.
- If you want to use herbs for something more specific, such as taking care of your skin, then consider planting: lavender, red clover, Roman camomile, myrtle, and calendula.

If your garden is already established, the herbs will need to fit into its existing layout. Check where there is room to plant your herbs, and whether the spaces are in light or shade, as this will influence the plants you might choose.

If you are starting an herb garden from scratch, then find the sunniest, warmest, and most sheltered part of your garden, because most culinary and medicinal herbs will thrive there.

Herb choices for full sun—*Dill, tarragon, fennel, hyssop, bay, lavender, oregano, cilantro, basil, sweet marjoram, rosemary, sage, and myrtle.*
These Mediterranean aromatic herbs have special cells within their leaves

that contain volatile oils—highly concentrated fragrances. The more sun these plants get, the stronger their aromas will be.

Herb choices for partial sun and partial shade—*Angelica, chervil, parsley, peppermint, sorrel, comfrey, wild strawberry, echinacea, eyebright, and Lady's mantle.*

These herbs grow best in dappled sunlight, out of the glare of full sun. In the wild their natural habitat is often at the edges of woods, where the canopy of trees is less dense, but still offers protection.

Herbs for full shade—*St. John's wort, evening primrose, lungwort, valerian, and sweet violet.*

These herbs do not need full sunlight, and tend to have rich green leaves.

A SIMPLE HERB GARDEN LAYOUT

One of the easiest herb gardens to create is a 10 ft (3 m) square, marked by a border of stones or bricks. Lay paving stones in a checkerboard pattern within the square, leaving bare squares of soil in between. Plant different herbs in each soil space; the paving stones let you step between them for easy picking.

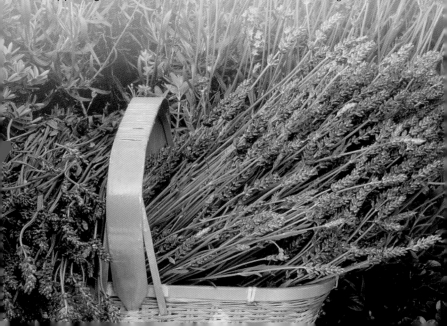

BELOW: Lavender, a Mediterranean aromatic herb, requires full sun to ensure a strong aroma

HARVESTING AND PROCESSING HERBS

Once they are established, many herbs are available all year round. Evergreens such as rosemary or myrtle will survive the winter, but the flavor and effect of their leaves will be much less intense in the colder months than in the summer, when their volatile oil content is highest. As such, it makes sense to identify the optimum time to harvest your herbs, when both their aromatic and therapeutic properties will be at their peak. With climate change currently occurring on a global scale, it is not possible to give definitive harvesting times for all regions—shorter winters and warmer spring seasons are bringing many plants into flower earlier than previously. You have to observe and smell your herbs to know when you should collect them—use the profile information on page 295 as a guide.

All herbs and flowers are best harvested on a dry day, ideally in the morning, before the sun has affected the plant. Use a sharp knife, scissors, or secateurs, choosing one species at a time, and gently lay the items flat in a basket. Pick out any weeds or damaged leaves, and ensure that the specimens are perfect. If you do not have much space to store herbs, then only pick a small amount.

BELOW: Herbs tied and hung should dry in about a week

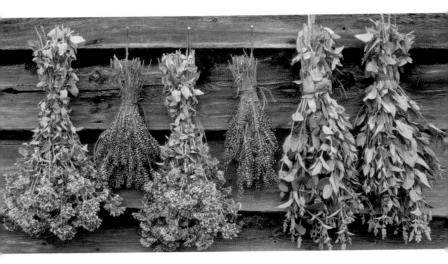

DRYING HERBS

Tie herbs like rosemary, sage, or thyme into small bunches and hang them upside down in a warm linen closet—they should dry in a week or so. Soft-stemmed herbs such as Lady's mantle, or flowers such as camomile can be laid individually on muslin on top of a cake cooling rack so that air circulates freely around them. If you do not have a linen closet you can place a tray or bunches of herbs tied together directly into a very cool oven at 90°F (33°C) and leave the oven door ajar overnight.

It is advisable to dry seeds in brown paper bags kept at room temperature for 2–3 weeks, completely away from moisture.

Roots ought to be thoroughly washed and wiped, and then tied together in bunches to hang up, or chopped into manageable pieces and dried on a tray.

ABOVE: Roots should be properly washed and wiped prior to drying

Leaves are ready when they become brittle, flowers when they are like tissue paper, and roots should snap easily when you bend them. Once your herbs are properly dried, store them in clean glass jars, clearly labeled with the contents. It is best to keep them out of direct sunlight in a cool, dark place. They will last for one year.

FREEZING HERBS

This works well for delicate leaves like basil, dill, fennel or chervil. Select small sprigs of each herb, place them in plastic bags and then freeze them. Alternatively, make aromatic ice cubes by placing chopped melissa or pepper-mint leaves in your ice cube trays.

SEASONAL HARVESTING

Late spring: angelica leaves and stems, borage leaves, chervil leaves, fennel leaves

Early summer: basil leaves, calendula flowers, elder flowers, sage leaves

Midsummer: angelica seeds, camomile flowers, lavender flowers, mint leaves

Late summer: bay leaves, dill seeds, elder berries, fennel seeds, garlic bulbs

Early fall: angelica root and dandelion root

WATER-BASED HERBAL PREPARATIONS

The easiest way to use herbs is to infuse them in boiling water to draw out their beneficial properties. Inhalations or face treatments use fragrant steam containing micro-droplets of volatile oils to help breathing or to cleanse the skin. Soaking in a bath softens the upper skin layers, while the hot water releases key herb ingredients to be absorbed for pain relief.

CLASSIC WATER-BASED PREPARATIONS

Drinking herb teas is a healthy alternative to caffeine-rich drinks such as ordinary tea or coffee. Herb teas are now easily obtainable as commercially prepared herbal teabags.

Standard infusions—this is a dose equivalent to one commercial teabag. To make an infusion, add 1 teaspoon (5 g) dried herb or 2 teaspoons (10 g) fresh leaves/flowers to a mug, then add 9 fl oz (250 ml) boiling water and leave to stand for 5 minutes. Add a teaspoon (5 ml) of honey to sweeten if you wish. As an example, 1 teaspoon (5 ml) of dried fennel seeds makes a lovely, refreshing, digestive tonic infusion.

Strong infusions are useful as wound-cleansing or skin-soothing remedies, or as rinses to promote shiny, healthy hair. When they have cooled, they can be used as compresses to help heal bruises or sprains. Put 2 teaspoons (10 g) dried herbs or 4 teaspoons (20 g) fresh leaves/flowers in a small bowl, add 9 fl oz (250ml) hot water, and allow to stand for 20 minutes. Try infusing 4 teaspoons (20 g) of fresh rosemary leaves in 9 fl oz (250 ml) water to make a revitalizing rinse for dark hair.

LEFT: Infusions can be used to treat a number of conditions

RIGHT: Herbal baths can both relax and invigorate, while also cleansing the skin

DECOCTIONS

These are made from dried roots, wood, or berries. Put 2 teaspoons (10 g) dried root/wood/berries in a small saucepan with 9 fl oz (250 ml) water; simmer the water for at least 15 minutes because the tough material takes longer to soften and release its ingredients. Two teaspoons (10 g) of dried angelica root makes a strong, bitter digestive tonic; take 2 teaspoons (10 ml) as one therapeutic dose.

FACIAL STEAMS/INHALATIONS

Boiling water with added leaves or flowers releases fragrant steam to deep cleanse the skin or ease blocked sinuses. Pour 30 fl oz (1 l) boiling water into a heatproof dish and set on a table. Scatter your herbs into the water, sit and lean over the steam with a towel over your head, and inhale for 10–15 minutes.

To deep cleanse the skin (weekly treatment):

3 tablespoons (45 g) fresh Roman camomile flowers

To clear the sinuses (morning and evening treatment):

3 tablespoons (45 g) fresh eucalyptus leaves

BATHS

Herbal baths cleanse the skin, as well as easing aches and pains. Put your chosen herbs in a small muslin bag hanging over the hot water tap as you fill the bath; they continue to infuse while you bathe. Therapeutic baths can be relaxing or invigorating—soak for 20 minutes for maximum effects. Try adding 2 fl oz (60 ml) full-cream milk to soften the water.

Relaxing baths

3 tablespoons (45 g) fresh lemon balm/melissa leaves

or 3 tablespoons (45 g) fresh sweet marjoram leaves

Invigorating baths

3 tablespoons (45 g) fresh heather flowering stems

or 3 tablespoons (45 g) fresh sage leaves

OIL-BASED HERBAL PREPARATIONS

In oil-based herbal preparations, a fatty base dissolves and draws out active ingredients from the herbs. Oil preparations are used for skin care, pain relief, or wound healing. One type—"macerated oil"—is easily applied with massage. Another is ointment, where oil is blended with wax and water to make a stable compound—this treats small areas of skin damage, such as cuts or grazes, or can be used for skin care.

MACERATED OILS

These are made with good-quality vegetable oil, gently heated with herbs to make aromatic preparations, excellent for aching muscles as well as dry skin. They are very easy to make.

EQUIPMENT

A medium, heavy-bottomed saucepan and lid

A heatproof glass bowl which sits inside the pan resting on the rim, without touching the bottom

A clean dark glass bottle, at least 8 oz (225 ml) capacity

INGREDIENTS

8 fl oz (225 ml) sunflower oil—you can use olive oil but it does have quite a strong aroma of its own

A generous handful of fresh herbs, for example, calendula and lavender flowers to calm and nourish the skin

Pour water into the saucepan to a depth of 1 in (2.5 cm) and heat until simmering; keep the heat low. Pour the oil into the heatproof bowl and add the flowers, making sure they are covered. Place the dish inside the saucepan over the simmering water, cover with the saucepan lid and leave over a low heat for one hour. Check the saucepan does not boil dry. Lift out the heatproof dish and allow to cool, then strain the oil into a jug, and carefully pour into the bottle. It will keep for 4–6 weeks.

Try these herb combinations:

Marjoram and myrtle leaves to ease menstrual pain

Heather flowers and comfrey leaves to help ease painful arthritis

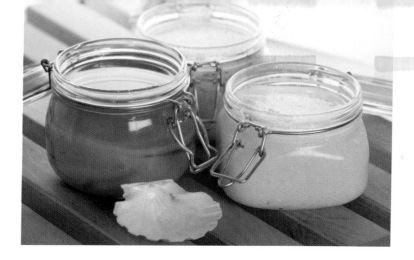

OINTMENTS

These thick, oil-based formulae have been made for thousands of years—the ancient Egyptians

ABOVE: Ointments have been used for thousands of years, for a variety of treatments

infused them with myrrh, frankincense, and spices. Making herbal ointment is like making mayonnaise the old-fashioned way; you just need to be patient while beating in the oil!

To make one 4 oz (120 g) pot of ointment:

EQUIPMENT

A small, heavy-bottomed saucepan

A heatproof glass bowl which sits inside the pan, resting on the rim without touching the bottom

A small metal whisk

A clean, dark brown glass jar with a screwtop lid (4 oz/120 g size)

INGREDIENTS

1 tablespoon (15 g) grated beeswax or
1 tablespoon (15 g) cocoa butter

4 tablespoons (60 ml) pre-prepared strong herbal infusion, such as comfrey, calendula, or camomile

4 tablespoons (60 ml) sunflower oil or
4 tablespoons (60 ml) of pre-prepared macerated oil for a stronger ointment

Pour cold water to cover the bottom of the saucepan up to 1 in (2.5 cm), and heat until simmering; keep the heat low. Add the infusion and the grated beeswax/cocoa butter to the heatproof bowl, then place the bowl inside the saucepan over the simmering water and whisk the mixture until the fat has dissolved. Then start whisking in the oil, just a few drops at a time; keep beating vigorously. When you have used all the oil, remove the dish from the heat and continue beating until the mixture thickens as it cools. Pour into the jar, seal and refrigerate. The ointment has an 8-week shelf life.

Some ointment ingredient combinations to try:

Macerated myrrh oil with calendula infusion for wound healing

Macerated red clover oil with myrtle leaf infusion for spots or acne

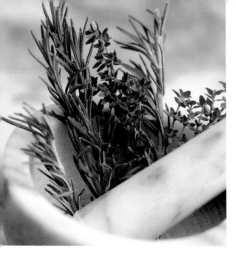

ALCOHOL-BASED HERBAL PREPARATIONS

Alcohol is the most efficient base to use for drawing out and preserving the active ingredients in herbs. Alcohol-based remedies remain potent for several years if they are stored tightly closed in a cool, dark place. They are only used in small quantities—a 1 fl oz (30ml) bottle of tincture will last for several weeks because just 20 drops diluted in water equals a single therapeutic dose.

TINCTURES

Tinctures are the most commonly used alcohol-based remedy. They have been in use for hundreds of years; the name comes from the Latin word "*tingere*," meaning "to dye." Alcohol draws pigments out of the plant material, giving the remedy a dark color. Many commercial herb tinctures are readily available in health-food stores and chemists, but you can make your own with good-quality brandy or vodka as a base.

Common herbs for tinctures

Echinacea for immune support

Red clover for skin and hormonal support

St. John's wort for stress

Sage for menopausal support

To make a tincture

Take 4 tablespoons (60 g) herb, bruise it slightly in a pestle and mortar, and place it in a large, dark glass jar or bottle (at least 10 floz/300 ml capacity). Pour over 10 fl oz (300 ml) either brandy or vodka, making sure all the herb is covered. Close the jar or bottle well and leave in a cool, dark place. Shake the bottle daily and after three weeks, strain the liquid thoroughly. Decant the tincture into dark glass bottles (the best kind to get have a rubber teat lid and a glass pipette inside, making it easy to extract drops; they can usually be obtained from pharmacists), and store in a cool, dark, dry place.

It is best to take tinctures on an empty stomach, just before meals. The adult dose is 20 drops (1 ml) of tincture in a small glass of water two to three times daily; children aged 10–15, ten drops; and children aged 5–9, five drops. Tinctures are not recommended for infants or babies.

FLOWER REMEDIES

These are another type of plant remedy preserved in alcohol. They were invented by Dr. Edward Bach in the early 20th century, as a way of using native wild plants and trees in homeopathic-like potencies to treat emotional and psychological problems such as fear, anger, shock, stubbornness, weariness, or melancholy.

The Bach method involves placing flowers or leaves on the surface of a bowl of spring water in strong direct sunlight; after a while the water is said to be "potentized" with the energetic frequency of the plant. The water is strained and preserved in equal parts of brandy to make a "mother stock," which is then used to make bottles of remedy.

The Bach flower healing system comprises 38 individual remedies and also includes a "rescue remedy" made up of five plants; this is used for acute emotional shock and distress. Flower remedies are now sold throughout the world, and new ones are being made from native plants in countries including Australia and the United States. The best way to take flower remedies is to drink six drops in a glass of water three times daily (this is suitable for adults or children over the age of five; they are not recommended for infants).

RIGHT: Flower remedies are used to treat a wide range of emotional problems

MUSCULAR ACHES AND FATIGUE

Our musculoskeletal system is made up of the skeleton and the muscular tissue which attaches to it. A healthy musculoskeletal system depends not just on good posture and exercise, but also on diet and metabolism—how efficiently our body transforms the foods and drinks we consume to repair, rebuild, and protect itself.

The skeleton is the body's support. It is made up of bone, cartilage, and bone marrow, where our red blood cells are formed. Joints—where two or more bones meet—are held together by pads of cartilage and ligaments; some of them are almost fixed, such as the joints between the bones in the skull, and others move freely, such as the shoulder or the knee.

Muscles attach to bones and help us to move. The body contains around 640 muscles, and they account for about half of our body weight. Two kinds exist in the body—voluntary muscles, which we are aware of, such as those we use for walking, and involuntary muscles, such as the bands around the large intestine, which are not under conscious control but enable elimination. Nerve impulses from the brain stimulate muscle fibers to contract and function. Muscle movement generates heat in the body and helps the circulation.

HOW HERBS HELP THE MUSCULOSKELETAL SYSTEM

Anti-rheumatics such as yarrow help ease rheumatic pain and discomfort.
Circulatory stimulants such as rosemary help improve blood supply to the muscles.
Mineral tonics such as horsetail are rich in silica which helps support bone formation.
Cleansing herbs such as nettle help eliminate toxins which can build up in muscle tissue.
Anti-inflammatory herbs such as comfrey help reduce swelling, particularly in the joints.

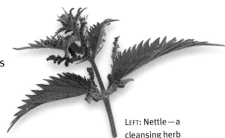

LEFT: Nettle—a cleansing herb

ABOVE: Macerated oils, combined with massage, make a good treatment for muscular aches and pains

MUSCULAR ACHES AND PAINS

Low-level mild aches and pains can be treated at home. However, if they persist you should consider consulting an osteopath or chiropractor to correct any underlying skeletal misalignments. Macerated oils (page 298) are very useful, applied using gentle massage to the affected area, with ingredients such as black pepper, rosemary, and juniper.

Pains due to injury, accidents, or trauma need medical assessment. First aid can be applied with herbs—cold compresses on injuries are helpful: use anti-inflammatory herbs such as German camomile, comfrey, or daisy to reduce swelling and relieve pain.

ARTHRITIS

It is important to know which type of arthritis you are addressing in order to select suitable herbs. If you are taking any anti-arthritic medication, always discuss the use of herbs with your doctor or a professional herbalist.

Osteoarthritis is caused by injury or by general wear and tear of the joints as the body ages, leading to stiffness, immobility, and muscular pain. Macerated oils (page 298) with circulatory stimulant herbs such as peppermint and ginger, or rosemary and eucalyptus, can be helpful.

Rheumatoid arthritis is an inflammatory response in the body linked to the immune system. The body is attacking its own tissues, particularly the lining of the joints, making them swollen and misshapen. Women are three times more likely to experience it than men. Try anti-inflammatory herbs such as German camomile, Devil's claw, or rose hip in capsules to ease pain.

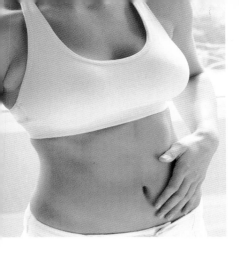

THE LIVER AND DIGESTION

The digestive tract is a long tube running through the body—it is around 25 ft (11 m) in length, and is lined with a moist membrane that secretes digestive juice to help the absorption of food. Our health depends on good digestive function—the foods we eat are full of nutrients we need to absorb to help our body repair and renew itself, as well as energy to fuel activity.

When we eat food, the teeth and saliva in the mouth help to reduce it to a smooth paste that we swallow into the stomach. In the small intestine more nutrients are absorbed. Bile, produced in the liver, and insulin from the pancreas help the process so that nutrients are absorbed into the blood. The body excretes waste products via the large intestine.

The movement of food through the system occurs because of muscular contractions that we do not consciously feel, however, digestive rhythm is very influenced by stress levels. Emotional tension often registers as interruptions or changes in bowel movement.

HOW HERBS HELP DIGESTION

Demulcents such as slippery elm soothe and protect the delicate digestive membrane. Bitters such as dandelion or German camomile stimulate the flow of bile from the liver.

Carminatives such as cinnamon or peppermint help ease wind in the gut.

Antispasmodics such as marjoram or melissa ease pain or spasm in the gut.

Tonics such as angelica or yellow gentian increase digestive juices.

Relaxants such as bitter orange help to soothe emotional stress linked to digestive problems.

RIGHT: Herbs can be used
to treat a huge variety of
digestive complaints

COMMON DIGESTIVE PROBLEMS

Indigestion is a combination of feelings of bloating, heaviness, or dull pain
after eating. Infusions of peppermint, fennel, or dill all contain volatile oils that
help counteract over-acidity and settle the digestion. If indigestion is due to
emotional stress, drink an infusion of lavender flowers.

Constipation occurs when the normal elimination is interrupted due to
factors such as an over-sedentary lifestyle or emotional stress. The bowel
should normally empty itself at least once a day, but constipation interferes
with this pattern so the abdomen becomes bloated and bowel movements
cause straining, pain and sometimes rectal bleeding. Any signs of bleeding
need medical attention.If there is a total blockage, senna provides quick relief,
but should not be used often. Infusions of herbs such as fennel or raspberry
leaf soothe the digestive tract more gently. If the condition is stress-related,
try German camomile or melissa infusions.

Irritable Bowel Syndrome (IBS) is a condition in which there are alternating
bouts of constipation and diarrhoea, sometimes with mucus in the feces and
varying levels of pain in the abdomen. Herbs can help to
re-establish normal bowel rhythm and reduce spasm
in the gut. Peppermint infusion is very soothing:
peppermint essential oil is also available in
capsules to be taken internally, so its antispasmodic effect soothes the intestinal wall.
Other useful herbs for infusions are fennel
and ginger.

The **liver** is vital to our health, and is the major
detoxifying organ of the whole body. Traditional
herbal medicine supports the liver with herbs such
as nettle or dandelion—in spring, infusions of young
leaves will cleanse and regulate liver
function. Bitter tonics such as yellow
gentian also support the liver.

RIGHT: Dandelion
is a traditional tonic
for the liver

IMMUNE AND RESPIRATORY FUNCTION

The immune system protects the body from invading micro-organisms such as bacteria, viruses, parasites, and fungi. We touch them and inhale them all the time. Mostly, if our immune systems are healthy, we are unaware of them. We only notice their presence when signs of illness demonstrate that the immune system cannot control them. The immune system is also affected by our moods and energy levels—high levels of stress, emotional upset, and physical tiredness will reduce the production of defensive cells, making us more likely to succumb to an infection.

The respiratory system is often where immune-related conditions take hold because of the constant ebb and flow of air out of the nose, throat, sinuses, windpipe, and lungs. The whole of the respiratory tract is lined with a mucus membrane that keeps the surfaces moist; in many respiratory conditions, too much mucus is produced and the body tries to get rid of it by coughing.

HOW HERBS CAN HELP

Immune tonics such as echinacea and garlic boost natural defenses.

Anti-microbials such as manuka and thyme destroy micro-organisms.

Adrenal tonics like cardamom and rosemary boost the body during recovery.

Expectorants such as white horehound and mullein help soothe coughs.

LEFT: The respiratory system is often a first point of contact with viruses and bacteria, and can be particularly susceptible to infection

COMMON IMMUNE PROBLEMS

Colds are caused by a range of viruses which lead to sneezing, stuffy heads, sore throats, and running noses. A traditional herbal combination for a cold is an infusion of equal parts yarrow, peppermint, and elderflower, which can be drunk four times daily. A hot infusion of 1 teaspoon (5 g) finely chopped fresh ginger with a slice of lemon and 1 teaspoon (5 ml) manuka honey can be taken three times daily to soothe sore throats and strengthen the respiratory system.

Catarrh is caused by overproduction of mucus and can lead to congestion and discomfort. Infusions of camomile, peppermint or elderflower help to tone the mucus membrane and loosen mucus. A steam inhalation with three drops of eucalyptus and three drops of rosemary essential oils will also ease chesty coughs.

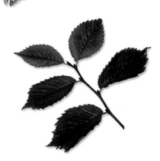

Sinusitis is an infection of the cavities inside the head, causing extreme pain in the cheeks and face. Tincture of echinacea taken three times daily, or an infusion of peppermint and thyme combined, helps the immune system as well as easing inflammation. Try taking garlic capsules daily to boost immune support.

Influenza is a viral infection in which the body experiences stabbing pains, shivers, and total loss of energy. An episode of flu will last about 7–10 days, and total bed rest is advised. Appetite will be low, but lots of fluids are needed—add honey and fresh lemon to infusions to help boost energy levels. Fresh ginger tea warms the body and supports the immune system, as does cardamom; a spicy infusion of these two is very refreshing. Echinacea tincture is advised three times daily.

ABOVE: Ginger (top) and slippery elm (bottom) are used to treat the immune system

Convalescence After periods of immune depletion, recovery can be supported by including slippery elm or oats in the diet to build strength in the body, and by eating manuka honey—a well-known immune-boosting food.

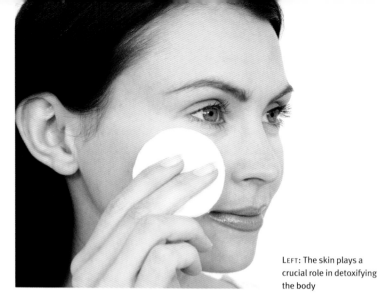

HERBS FOR HEALTHY SKIN

308 **The skin is a supple and sensitive surface enabling us to touch, sense, and
feel our world. It regulates our temperature via sweat released through
special glands. The skin is sometimes called the "third kidney" because it
plays such an important role in detoxifying the body.**

The skin has three main layers. The epidermis is the outer layer made up of
layers of cells containing a protective ingredient called keratin, also found in
our hair and nails. Below, the dermis contains a network of fine blood vessels,
sensory nerve receptors, sweat glands, hair follicles, and sebaceous glands
that secrete lubrication onto the surface to keep the epidermis supple. The
lowest layer is the subcutaneous fat that conserves body heat.

HOW HERBS HELP THE SKIN

Cleansers such as red clover and nettle detoxify impurities.
Anti-inflammatories such as camomile and comfrey soothe soreness.
Vulneraries such as horsetail and myrrh promote wound healing.
Anti-microbials such as thyme and echinacea fight infection.
Cytophylactics such as lavender and myrtle promote healthy skin growth.
Diuretics such as yarrow and nettle eliminate waste products via the kidneys.

TYPICAL SKIN PROBLEMS

For **cuts and wounds,** cleanse the area with a strong antiseptic infusion of horsetail or yarrow to stop excessive bleeding. If infection is present, hot compresses of anti-microbials such as thyme or garlic 2–3 times daily will help draw out matter. Applying ointment containing herbs such as calendula or comfrey 2–3 times daily will help the wound heal cleanly.

Acne is where a series of red pustules with yellow pus appear on the face, neck, shoulders, or back. The sebaceous glands become blocked and inflamed, often as a result of hormonal imbalance, but also due to poor diet and elimination. The skin needs cleansing and toning with witch-hazel extract to help fight infection. Ointment with red clover or calendula can help reduce infection and heal the lesions.

Boils are localized infected areas swollen with a bacterial infection. Apply hot compresses twice daily using strong infusions of myrtle or echinacea to help to draw out matter. Apply ointment containing calendula or comfrey twice daily to speed up healing.

ABOVE: Camomile is a popular treatment for conditions like eczema

Eczema is often a stress-related condition or linked to dietary allergies to sugar, wheat, or dairy products. Small lesions break open into reddish weeping areas, particularly between fingers or in creases or folds of skin. After a while the skin may become hard and scaly as the epidermis thickens to try and protect itself. Cooled, strong, German camomile infusion or aloe vera gel can be applied as needed to calm irritation. Soothing and skin-repairing ointment combinations such as red clover and calendula can be applied to repair damaged areas, especially at night to allow time for it to work.

Psoriasis is when large patches of the lower epidermal layer become exposed too soon, shedding silvery skin cells and exposing red, inflamed areas, often found on the elbows or knees. Macerated oil with lavender flowers and comfrey is extremely soothing when applied externally; another good combination of skin-calming herbs would be calendula and red clover.

ABOVE: Horsetail—a strong antiseptic for treating wounds

THE NERVOUS SYSTEM

The nervous system is a complex communication network that passes electrical messages between the brain and the rest of the body. The nervous system responds to changing levels of stress—modern life can cause it to be constantly over-triggered into what is called "fight or flight" mode. Anxieties, pressures, deadlines, traveling, rushing food, or skipping meals can all stretch the body's ability to cope. Sleep problems, recurring immune infections, digestive upsets, and mood swings are common signs of nervous system imbalance.

Long-term chronic stress can have severely depleting effects on the body—the immune response is lowered, and the body's ability to fight infections becomes compromised. Viral infections can lead to conditions known as "post-viral fatigue," "chronic fatigue syndrome," or ME (*myalgic encephalomyelitis*), where the body struggles to recover normal levels of energy. Plenty of rest and treatment with herbs can be very beneficial to recovery.

HOW HERBS HELP THE NERVOUS SYSTEM

Nerve restoratives such as oats and borage nourish the nervous system.

Sedatives such as camomile and bitter orange promote relaxation and sleep.

Stimulants such as ginseng and rosemary can relieve tiredness and increase energy.

Immune-boosting herbs such as garlic and echinacea rebuild the body's defenses.

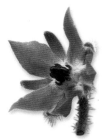

ABOVE: Borage is an excellent restorative for the nervous system

COMMON NERVE-RELATED PROBLEMS

Headaches often occur as a sign of mental stress or eye strain. Standard infusions of peppermint or German camomile can relieve pain, or essential oil of lavender can be applied neat to the forehead (2 drops maximum) as an analgesic. If you suffer repeatedly from headaches, consult your doctor.

Migraines are severe, one-sided headaches that can send violent pain down the face, and cause visual disturbances and nausea. Feverfew is a good

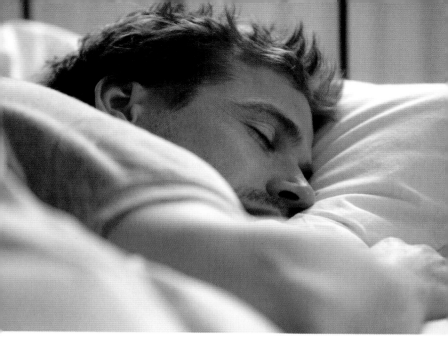

remedy for migraines. Standard infusions of herbs such as peppermint or valerian are pain-killing and relieve nausea. Avoid migraine-triggering foods such as cheese, chocolate, red wine, or high levels of sugar. If symptoms persist, seek medical advice.

Low mental energy can be caused by long-term mental stress. Passion flower capsules or tincture restore the nervous system, and St. John's wort or borage capsules ease anxiety or depression. While ginseng can increase energy, consider lifestyle changes to help ease underlying stress patterns.

Persistent fatigue caused by long-term mental stress can lead to "post-viral fatigue" or ME. In these cases, it is best to seek treatment from a professional herbalist. However, it is beneficial to drink infusions of sedative herbs such as sweet marjoram or melissa to help sleep. Echinacea tincture boosts immune function, and oat tincture eases chronic stress levels. Infusions of cleansing herbs such as nettle or red clover detoxify the blood and lymphatic system. Eating oats helps to rebuild physical strength.

Insomnia Sleep problems can arise due to an inability to switch off at the end of the day, from eating heavy meals, or drinking caffeine-rich drinks late at night. Infusion of lavender or passion flower reduces tension before bed. Capsules of valerian or melissa can be taken to improve relaxation.

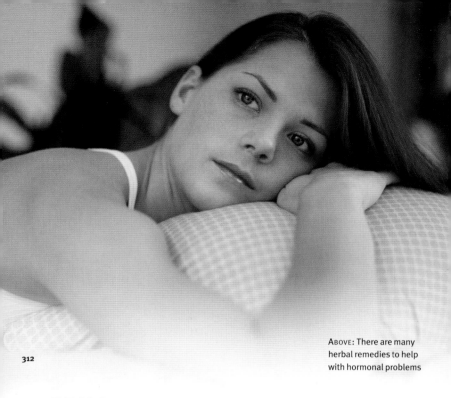

ABOVE: There are many herbal remedies to help with hormonal problems

FEMALE HORMONAL SUPPORT

Hormones are chemical messengers that are sent by the brain to influence processes in the body. In many cultures herbs have been used to support female hormonal issues. Scientific research has now identified ingredients called plant sterols that occur in many traditional hormone-support herbs — they are similar to our own human hormones, which explains their beneficial effects.

A WOMAN'S HORMONAL LIFE

At around the age of 12, girls begin to menstruate. The menstrual cycle starts on the first day of bleeding, and by days 14–16 the lining of the womb has thickened and an egg has been released. If the egg is not fertilized, the lining of the womb will degenerate and be lost as the menstrual flow. If the egg is fertilized, the lining thickens as the embryo embeds itself and starts growing into a baby.

In pregnancy, use of herbs should always be supervised by a professional herbalist, because many herbs can cause menstrual bleeding or stimulate the womb. During labor, herbs such as raspberry leaf can be used to help maintain the frequency of contractions.

From approximately the age of 45, the frequency of menstruation slows and hormonal changes take place until it ceases. This is the menopause.

HOW HERBS HELP FEMALE HORMONE PROBLEMS

Astringents such as yarrow and nettle regulate excess menstrual bleeding.

Antispasmodics such as lavender and German camomile can ease cramps.

Emmenagogues such as cinnamon and ginger stimulate menstrual flow, particularly if it is scanty or absent. It must be established that the woman is not pregnant before using them.

Hormone regulators such as agnus castus and black cohosh balance the female sex hormones during menstruation or the menopause.

Nerve tonics such as melissa and St. John's wort help to calm mood swings.

Uterine tonics such as Lady's mantle and raspberry leaf strengthen the womb.

ABOVE: Cinnamon can help to stimulate menstrual flow

COMMON PROBLEMS

Pre-Menstrual Syndrome (PMS) includes symptoms such as mood swings, temporary weight increase, abdominal bloating or headaches, which are experienced during the latter part of the menstrual cycle. Drinking an infusion of Lady's mantle or raspberry leaf can help to raise energy levels. Regular supplementation with evening primrose oil for at least four months greatly improves PMS symptoms.

Irregular or painful periods are a sign of hormone imbalance. Any sudden change in menstrual rhythm or flow should be discussed with your phyiscian, particularly if the periods stop. Drinking an infusion of Lady's mantle regularly or taking agnus castus tincture or black cohosh capsules can help to regulate period length and frequency.

Menopausal symptoms include headaches, hot flushes, heart palpitations, mood swings, insomnia, and low libido—all due to changing hormone levels. Herbs with estrogen-like effects include agnus castus and black cohosh. Yarrow infusion can help night sweats or hot flushes. A proper menopause support programme should be supervised by a professional herbalist.

MALE HORMONAL SUPPORT

The ancient traditional medicine of China and India places great emphasis on the sexual and hormonal health of the male, using herbs to strengthen and tone the reproductive organs. In the West, interest in these approaches is increasing due to the debilitating effects of stress many men experience in daily life. Persistent physical and emotional pressure can cause problems such as low sperm count and impotence. In later life, many men also experience problems relating to the prostate gland. Fortunately, many herbs have beneficial toning and restorative effects on male physiology.

THE ORGANS OF MALE REPRODUCTION

The testes produce sperm and secrete testosterone, the male sex hormone, which is responsible for bone and muscle growth, and sexual development.
The scrotum is the sac that contains the testes. It allows sperm to develop at a lower temperature outside of the body.

BELOW: Herbs can be used to treat the many effects of stress

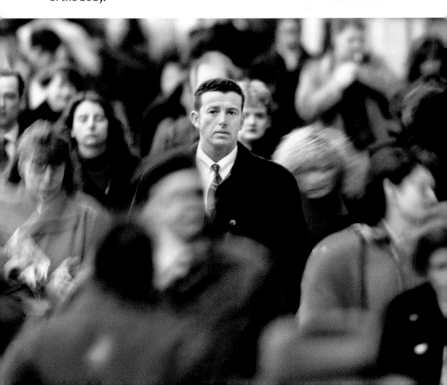

The penis is the male sex organ through which semen (sperm swimming in fluid) and urine pass.

The prostate gland is about the size of a walnut, situated under the bladder. It produces the fluids that are mixed with sperm during ejaculation. It grows to full size during puberty. Due to changing hormone levels, in many men it can enlarge after the age of 50, causing urinary problems and sometimes cancer.

HOW HERBS SUPPORT MALE HORMONAL FUNCTION

Adrenal tonics such as ginseng and damiana can help to relieve exhaustion and increase energy.

Tonics such as ginger and saw palmetto energize the sexual organs and strengthen sexual function.

Urinary tonics such as saw palmetto and horsetail fern support the action of the prostate gland.

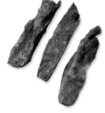

COMMON PROBLEMS

Impotence is a man's inability to achieve or sustain an erection. It is often a symptom of underlying problems such as worry, stress, or low energy levels. Tonic herbs such as ginger, ginseng, or damiana, taken as either

ABOVE: Ginseng is a powerful restorative for increasing energy levels

supplements or infusions, can renew energy levels and tone the reproductive system. Lifestyle changes also need to be considered.

Prostate enlargement is a common condition affecting one in three males over the age of 50. Due to hormonal fluctuations the prostate gland can enlarge, causing it to press on the bladder, which causes a frequent need to pass urine. However the pressure of the enlargement can cause a reduction in the stream of urine so the bladder does not feel completely empty. Saw palmetto capsules can be taken daily, or infusions of tonic herbs such as horsetail fern and nettle can be drunk 2–3 times daily to help restore flow. The condition should also be monitored by a doctor.

Prostatitis is a bacterial infection in the prostate which needs medical support. The symptoms are: fever, lower back pain and burning on urination. Infusions of antiseptic herbs such as thyme, anti-inflammatories such as German camomile, or diaphoretics such as elderflower taken 2–3 times daily reduce fever and pain. Echinacea tincture can be taken to support the immune system. Any unusual lower abdominal pain or swelling should be referred to your physician.

GLOSSARY

Active ingredient—a medicinally active substance

Acute—a condition which comes on rapidly and intensively, and is of short duration

Alkaloid—strong-acting plant ingredient

Anemia—deficiency of iron

Analgesic—reduces pain

Anaphrodisiac—reduces sexual desire

Antibiotic—kills micro-organisms

Anti-inflammatory—reduces inflammation

Antirheumatic—eases rheumatism

Antispasmodic—relieves spasm of involuntary muscles (e.g., colon)

Antiseptic—kills bacterial micro-organisms

Annual—a plant with a single-year life cycle, requiring fresh sowing each year

Aphrodisiac—increases sexual desire

Aromatic—a substance with a fragrant scent

Astringent—contracts tissue and stops bleeding

Bark—the outer covering of a woody stem or trunk

Biennial—a plant that completes its life cycle in two years, growing in year 1 and flowering or fruiting in year 2

Bitter—a substance that is usually antibacterial and bitter tasting

Bulb—an underground storage organ with fleshy leaves and a short stem around next year's shoot

Carminative—relieves intestinal gas

Chronic—a condition with milder symptoms but persisting over a long period

Compress—a wet pad of material applied to areas of the body

Compound—(of leaves or flowers) meaning a cluster with branches

Decoction—a preparation of roots or tough plant material boiled in water

Deciduous—a tree or shrub that drops its leaves each fall and re-grows them in spring

Demulcent—a soothing substance that protects mucus membranes

Diaphoretic—increases perspiration

Digestive tonic—helps digestive processes

Dioecious—a plant species in which the male and female flowers grow on separate plants

Diuretic—increases elimination of water via the kidneys and bladder

Edema—build-up of fluid in the tissues

Emmenagogue—stimulates menstruation

Essential oil—a concentrated fragrant essence distilled from a single plant

Evergreen—a tree or shrub that retains its leaves all year round

Expectorant—helps the chest expel excess phlegm

Fatty oil—a natural vegetable oil e.g., evening primrose

Flavonoid—a group of organic pigments in plants

Galactogogue—stimulates breast-milk flow

Glycoside—a substance containing sugar

Hybrid—a plant produced by crossing two species (shown with an *x* in the Latin name)

Indigenous—a plant native to the place where it grows

Infusion—plant material steeped in boiling water

Introduced—a plant species brought to an area by man

Macerated oil—a therapeutic remedy where herbs are infused in oil and heated

Mucilage—a gel-like substance secreted by certain plants

Ointment—an oil- and fat-based emulsion used to heal the skin

Perennial—a plant that lives for more than two years

Rhizome—a fleshy root, e.g., ginger

Rubefacient—has a localized reddening effect on the skin

Runners—a creeping root system

Saponins—plant ingredients that foam in water

Sedative—a calming substance that relieves tension and causes drowsiness

Stimulant—a substance that increases physiological activity

Tannins—a group of plant ingredients with astringent and antibacterial effects

Tap root—a thick, main root growing straight downward, e.g., carrot

Tincture—a plant remedy made by soaking material in alcohol

Tonic—an invigorating action on the body

Umbel—an umbrella shaped flower head with stalks of equal length radiating out from one point, e.g., angelica

Vulnerary—wound-healing action

Professional herbal associations:

American Herbalists Guild
141 Nob Hill Road, Cheshire
CT 06410 USA
Tel: 203 272 6731
www.americanherbalistsguild.com
Email: ahgoffice@earthlink.net

American Botanical Council
6200 Manor Rd, Austin, TX 78723, USA
Tel: 512 926 4900
www.herbalgram.org

The Herb Society of America
9019 Kirtland Chardon Road
Kirtland, OH 44094
Tel: 440 256 0514
www.herbsociety.org
Email: herbs@herbsociety.org

American Herb Association
PO Box 1673, Nevada City, CA 95959
www.ahaherb.com

American Herbal Products Association
8484 Georgia Ave., Suite 370
Silver Spring, MD 20910
Tel: 301 588 1171
www.ahpa.org
Email: ahpa@ahpa.org

Retailers:

Frontier Natural Products Co-op
PO Box 299 3021 78th St.
Norway, IA 52318
Tel: 800-669-3275
www.frontiercoop.com
Email: customercare@frontiercoop.com

INDEX

A

Abu Ibn Sina 6
Achillea millefolium 22
Aesculapius 64
Aesculus hippocastanum 24
Alchemilla vulgaris 26
Alkaloids 16
Allium sativum 28
Aloe vera 30
Anemone pulsatilla 32
Anethum graveolens 34
Angelica archangelica 36
Angelica polymorpha 38
Anthemis nobilis 40
Anthriscus cerefolium 42
Apium graveolens 44
Arctium lappa 46
Arctostaphylos uva ursi 48
Armoracia rusticana 50
Arnica montana 52
Artemisis dracunculus 54
Aspirin 16, 114, 218
Avena sativa 56
Ayurvedic medicine 6, 44, 76, 90, 100

B

Bach flower remedy system 204, 301
Bach, Dr Edward 301
Baths 19, 296
Bee balm see Melissa officinalis
Bellis perennis 58
Betula pendula 60
Bible, The 86, 144
Bitters 16
Bloodwort see Achillea millefolium
Borago officinalis 62
Brassica nigra 64
Bread and cheese tree see Crategus oxyacantha
Buttercup 74

C

Calendula officinalis 66
Candlewick plant see Verbascum thapsus
Capsicum frutescens 68
Captain Lewis 140
Carboniferous era, The 102
Cassia senna 70
Castenea vesca 24
Centaurea cyanus 72
Chasteberry see Vitex agnus castus
Chinese Angelica see Angelica sinensis
Cimifuga racemosa 74
Cinnamomum zeylanicum 76
Citrus aurantium 78
Citrus limonum 80
Citrus paradisi 82
Commiphora myrrha 84
Compresses 19
Coriandrum sativum 86
Crategus oxyacantha 88
Culpeper, Nicholas 22, 34, 42, 46, 54, 56, 62, 112, 144, 156, 164, 216, 228, 236, 244, 260
Curcuma longa 90
Cymbopogon citratus 92

D

Dang gui See Angelica sinensis
Daucus carota 94
Decoctions 19
Dioscorea villosa 96
Dioscorides 6, 32, 34, 144, 192
Dog rose see Rosa canina

E

Echinacea purpurea 98
Elephant thistle see Silybum marianum
Elettaria cardamomum 100
Elizabeth I 94
Equisetum arvense 102
Erica vulgaris 104

Erythrea centaurium 106
Eucalyptus globules 108
Eugenia caryophylla 110
Euphrasia officinalis 112
Evelyn, John 54

F

Facial steam 19, 296
Feverwort see Erythrea centaureum
Filipendula ulmaria 114
Flavonoids 17
Foeniculum vulgare 116
Fragaria vesca 118
Frankincense 84
Fucus vesiculosus 120

G

Galium verum 122
Gentiana lutea 124
Gerard, John 50, 56, 62, 68, 162, 174, 220
Gingko biloba 126
Glycosides 16
Glycyrrhiza glabra 128
Great Plague, The 36
Grieve see Mrs Grieve
Gum / Resin 16

H

Hamamelis virginiana 130
Harpogophytum procumbens 132
Helianthus annuus 134
Herbal tea 19, 34
Herodotus 28
Hieronymous Tragus 26
Hildegard of Bingen 56, 116
Hippocrates 6
Hippophae rhamnoides 136
Humulus lupulus 138
Hydrastis canadensis 140
Hypericum perforatum 142
Hyssopus officinalis 144

318